Cardiovascular English

Ramón Ribes · Sergio Mejía

Ramón Ribes · Sergio Mejía

Cardiovascular English

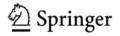 Springer

Ramón Ribes, MD, PhD
Hospital Reina Sofia
Servicio de Radiología
Avda. Menéndez Pidal s/n.
Córdoba 14004, Spain

Sergio Mejía, MD, PhD
Xanit International Hospital
Benalmádena, Spain

ISBN 978-3-540-73141-2   e-ISBN 978-3-540-73142-9

DOI 10.1007/978-3-540-73142-9

Library of Congress Control Number: 2007939514

© 2008 Springer-Verlag Berlin · Heidelberg

Cover design: Frido Steinen-Broo, eStudio Calamar, Spain

Printed on acid-free paper

9 8 7 6 5 4 3 2 1

springer.com

To my mother, Maribel Bautista Sierra,
my first teacher, for her endless love.

R. Ribes

To my children, from the bottom of my heart.

S. Mejía

Preface

After the successful publication of *Medical English, Radiological English and Primary Care English* by Springer, I considered it a top priority to keep on writing medical English books by specialties, which could become useful tools for health care professionals and medical students all over the world.

Being a cardiovascular radiologist myself, *Cardiovascular English* was one of the first titles that came to my mind when I began to think about a series of medical English books by specialties. In spite of the fact that cardiovascular diseases are my main area of interest, I would not have dared co-write a book on cardiovascular English without the enthusiastic support of Dr. Mejía.

This book project started in Benalmadena when, during the dinner after a 1-day course on cardiovascular imaging, Dr. Manuel Concha, a prominent figure in cardiac surgery and one of the pioneers of cardiac transplants in my country, and who was aware of my idea of writing a cardiovascular English book, introduced Dr. Mejía to me saying "Ramón, Sergio is the person you are looking for."

He was absolutely right. Sergio Mejía has been enthusiastically committed to the book project since its inception.

Like its predecessors, *Cardiovascular English* is not written by English teachers and aimed at English students, but it is written by doctors and aimed at doctors.

Dr. Mejía has done an excellent job, on the one hand, adapting to *Cardiovascular English* some of the chapters of both medical English and radiological English, and on the other hand, designing and writing *Cardiovascular English* chapters in which we try to help the non-native English-speaking cardiologist, cardiology resident, nurse, or medical student deal with the nuances of day-to-day cardiovascular English.

We are currently working on several book projects that we hope will become new titles of the series of medical English books by specialties, and look forward to your feedback in order to improve the series and provide health care professionals with more books aimed at other medical specialties in the future.

August 2007   Ramón Ribes, MD, PhD

Preface

More than two decades ago, we medical students at the Health Sciences Institute in Medellín, Colombia, listened astonished to our professors when they asked us to read our medical textbooks in English. It was a real challenge for a group of non-native English speakers, not only to study pathology, anatomy, and physiology, but to do it in English. "They are crazy," we thought. But nowadays, I really appreciate the importance of that idea. It was brilliant. They not only recommended us, but also did their best to send us to North American hospitals to do short rotations as visitors.

As a matter of fact, English is the language of science. If you want to be able to communicate with colleagues worldwide, and if you want to take advantage of using the Internet and keeping up to date, then you need a high level of mastery of the English language.

Some of you might think, "But if this author lives in Spain, what is he talking about?" Well, I work at an international hospital in southern Spain, the beach of Europe. Please take care and read carefully. I have written the "beach" of Europe. So we have many many visitors, tourists, and residents from Northern and Central Europe as our population of interest. In my hospital, we treat patients from Finland to Germany, and it is not possible to do a good job if you do not speak English.

When Dr. Ribes kindly invited me to co-write *Cardiovascular English*, I was delighted to have the opportunity to help non-native English-speaking colleagues to improve their cardiovascular English knowledge. This manual is part of a medical English series coordinated by Dr. Ribes, and I hope it will be very useful to those students, residents, nurses, technicians, and specialists who want to make some forward movement. Traveling, attending an international congress for the first time, submitting an abstract, writing an article, presenting a paper, attending a course abroad, and so on are all forward professional movements, especially when one is a non-native-English speaker.

I also want to acknowledge the cooperation of the contributors. They are of key importance in the final delivery of this book.

Western countries are looking at the Far East, and that will probably be the next step in globalization and part of the twenty-first century's history. In this process, English seems to be the common language, that is, the "second" language for everyone. Cardiovascular professionals are not the exception. So let us move forward and get involved in the adventure of learning English, getting used to cardiovascular English. Please enjoy the reading.

August 2007   Sergio Mejía, MD, PhD

Table of Contents

III Cardiological Scientific Literature: Writing an Article

IV Letters to Editors of Cardiovascular Journals

V Attending an International Cardiological Course

VI Giving a Cardiological Talk

VII Chairing a Cardiological Session

VIII Usual Mistakes Made by Cardiologists when Speaking and Writing In English

IX Latin and Greek Terminology

X Acronyms and Abbreviations

XI Cardiovascular Clinical History

XII Cardiovascular Examination

XIII Prescribing Medication

XIV Echocardiography

XV Invasive Cardiac Imaging: the Cath Lab

XVI Electrocardiogram Interpretation

XVII Heart Transplantation

XVIII Clinical Session

XIX On Call

XX Conversation Survival Guide

Contributors

PEDRO J. ARANDA
Servicio de Cirugía Cardiovascular
Hospital Universitario Carlos Haya
Málaga, Spain

FRANCISCO J. MUÑOZ DEL CASTILLO
ENT Consultant and Family Doctor
Reina Sofía University Hospital
Córdoba, Spain
(Drew the illustrations)

ELOISA FELIÚ
Radiologist
INSCANNER
Alicante, Spain

ANTONIO LUNA
Radiologist
SERCOSA
Jaén, Spain

JOSÉ MARÍA MARTOS
Radiologist
Puente Genil Hospital
Córdoba, Spain

JOSÉ LUIS SANCHO
Radiologist
Montilla Hospital
Córdoba, Spain

JOSÉ MARÍA VIDA
Radiologist
Montilla Hospital
Córdoba, Spain

UNIT I

Unit I Methodological Approach to Cardiovascular English

Introduction

The learning of cardiovascular English is one of the most demanding of all medical English by specialty. The multiplicity of cardiological subspecialties makes it extremely difficult to be familiar with the jargon of each subspecialty: A clinical cardiologist would be completely lost in a talk on arrhythmia ablation (arrhythmia itself is one of the most frequently misspelled medical words), and a sonographer might not know the name of most interventional cardiology devices.

How to be Fluent in Cardiological English

A sound knowledge of English grammar is pivotal in order to build your cardiovascular English consistently. To be fluent in anatomical English is crucial for cardiologists involved in cardiovascular imaging. Cardiologists need to know what the normal structures look like and are called, and how to express their relationships with radiological findings (although we cardiologists are not radiologists, we have at our disposal multiple imaging techniques for the study of the heart). Anatomy is so linked to Latin and Greek that unless you are familiar with Latin and Greek terminology, you will never be able to speak and write both anatomical and cardiovascular English properly. Besides, cardiologists must be aware of the technical aspects of their subspecialties and must be able to talk about them in an intelligible manner to patients, referring physicians, residents, nurses, technicians, and medical students.

Besides the technical medical language, the cardiologist must understand what we call the patients' "medical English," which is the language used by patients when talking about their conditions and the usual expressions used by patients with regard to their illnesses.

Let us do a simple exercise. Read this sentence of cardiological English:

"Kaplan-Meier survival estimates at 1 year for the respective occurrence of death, Q-wave MI, repeat CABG, and target lesion revascularization (TLR) were 90, 94, 96, and 76%, respectively, after stent implantation."

We are sure you understand the sentence and that you are able to translate it into your own language almost instantly; unfortunately, translation is not only useless, but it is also deleterious to your cardiological English with regard to fluency.

If you try to read the paragraph in English aloud, then your first difficulties will appear.

If a conversation on the sentence starts and the audience is waiting for your opinion, then you may begin to sweat.

If you are not familiar with statistics, then "Kaplan-Meier survival" may sound to you as the survival of two patients named Kaplan and Meier.

Check the words you are not able to pronounce easily and look them up in the dictionary.

Ask an English-speaking colleague to read it aloud; try to write it; probably you will find some difficulty in writing certain words.

Check the words you are not able to write properly and look them up in the dictionary.

Finally, try to have a conversation on the topic.

Notice how many problems have been raised by just one sentence of cardiological English. Our advice is that once you have diagnosed your actual cardiovascular English level:

- Do not get depressed if it is below your expectations.
- Keep on doing these exercises with progressively longer paragraphs, beginning with those belonging to your subspecialty.
- Arrange cardiovascular English sessions at your institution. A session once a week might be a good starting point. The sessions will keep you, and your colleagues, in touch with at least a weekly cardiovascular English meeting. You will notice that you feel much more confident talking to colleagues with a lower level than yours than talking to your native English teacher, as you will feel better talking to non-native English speaking cardiologists than talking to native English-speaking colleagues. In these sessions you can rehearse the performance of talks and lectures so that when you give a presentation at an international meeting it is not the first time it has been delivered.

Let us evaluate our cardiovascular English level with these ten simple (?) exercises.

Are the following sentences correct?

1. Pulsed and continuous Doppler techniques have provided the data that enhance the prospect of managing critically ill neonates noninvasively and without confirmatory cardiac catheterization.
   Not correct.

The use of "-wave" after pulsed and continuous is imperative, as we are always talking about the wave mode used when we register flow velocities with the Doppler machine. Therefore, the correct sentence is "Pulsed- and continuous-*wave* Doppler techniques have provided ..."

2. Later, it was showed that cigarette smoking produced silent ST segment depression.
   Not correct.

The correct sentence is "Later, it was *shown* that cigarette smoking produced silent ST-segment depression."

This is a very common mistake. The past participle of the verb *show* is not *showed* but *shown*. Being "showed" the past tense of the verb *show*, many health care professionals imply, erroneously, that it is a regular verb.

3. Syncope due to primary hypertension is often preceded of dizziness and faintness.
   Not correct.

The correct sentence is "Syncope due to primary hypertension is often preceded *by* dizziness and faintness."

The use of the appropriate preposition plays a vital role in medical English. Many mistakes of this sort are related to the use of the preposition, as if you were speaking in your own language. Do not forget to double-check prepositional verbs and prepositions whenever you write in English; most of the time these prepositions are not the same as in your native tongue.

4. A 38-years-old patient with heavy chest pain.
   Not correct.

The correct phrase is "38-year-old patient with heavy chest pain."

"38-year-old" is, in this case, an adjective, and adjectives when they precede a noun, cannot be written in the plural. Although extremely simple from a grammatical standpoint, this is, probably, the commonest mistake in international medical presentations.

5. There was not biopsy of the right ventricle.
   Not correct.

The correct sentence is "There was *no* biopsy of the right ventricle."

We could have said instead "there was not a biopsy of the right ventricle" or "there was not any biopsy of the right ventricle."

6. An 87-year-old patient with an arrythmia.
   Not correct.

The correct phrase is "87-year-old patient with an arr*h*ythmia."

Arrhythmia is one of the most commonly misspelled words in medical English. You can avoid this recurrent mistake by checking that the word "rhythm" (provided it is spelled correctly!) is embedded in "arrhythmia."

7. How would you ask a patient to perform a Valsalva maneuver?
   "Bear down (or push) as if you are having a bowel movement."

8. Are "Harvard students" and "Harvard alumni" synonymous?
   No.

The former term refers to current students and the latter to former students.

9. Are "home calls" and "in-house calls" synonymous?
   No.

They are not synonymous, but antonymous; they express opposite concepts. With "home calls" you will hopefully sleep at home, whereas with "in-house calls" you must stay in the hospital for the whole clinical duty.

10. What would you understand if in an interventional cardiology suite you hear "Dance with me?"
    Someone is asking to have his/her gown tied up.

This set of questions is intended for those who think that cardiovascular English is not worth to giving a second thought. On the one hand, most cardiologists and cardiovascular surgeons who have never worked in English-speaking hospitals tend to underestimate the difficulty of cardiovascular English; they think that provided you speak English, you will not find any problems in cardiological environments. However, those who have suffered embarrassing situations working abroad do not dare say that either English or cardiovascular English are easy.

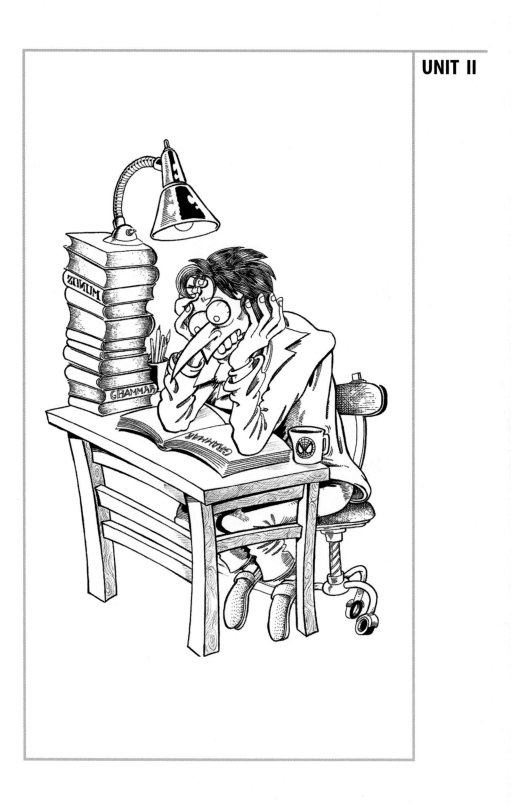

Unit II Cardiovascular Grammar

Introduction

The first chapters are probable the least read by most readers in general, but in our opinion, it is precisely in the first chapters that the most important information of a book is displayed. It is in the first chapters where the foundations of a book are laid, and many readers do not optimize the reading of a manual because they skip its fundamentals.

This is a vital chapter because unless you have a sound knowledge of English grammar, you will be unable to speak English as it is expected from a well-trained cardiologist. At your expected English level, it is definitely not enough just to be understood; you must speak fluently, and your command of the English language must allow you to communicate with your colleagues and patients, regardless of their nationality.

As you will see immediately, this grammar section is made up of cardiological sentences, so at the same time that you revise, for instance, the passive voice, you will be reviewing how to say usual sentences in day-to-day cardiological English such as "the 2D-echo scan had already been performed when the chairperson arrived at the non-invasive unit."

We could say, to summarize, that we have replaced the classic sentence of older English manuals, "My tailor is rich," by expressions such as "The first-year cardiology resident is on call today." Without a certain grammatical background, it is not possible to speak correctly, just as without certain knowledge of anatomy, it would not be possible to make a good cardiological practice nor report on cardiological examinations. The tendency to skip both grammar and anatomy, considered by many as simple preliminary issues, has had deleterious effects on the learning of English and cardiology.

Tenses

Talking about the Present

Present Continuous

The present continuous tense shows an action that is happening in the present time at or around the moment of speaking.

Present simple of the verb *to be* + gerund of the verb: *am/are/is ...-ing*.

Study this sample:

It is 7.30 in the morning. Dr. Smith is in his new car on his way to the Cardiology Department.

So, he *is driving* to the Cardiology Department, meaning that he is driving now, at the time of speaking.

USES

To talk about:

- Something that is happening at the time of speaking (i.e., now):

  - Dr. Hudson *is going* to the emergency room.
  - Dr. Smith's colleague *is performing* an angioplasty.

- Something that is happening around or close to the time of speaking, but not necessarily exactly at the time of speaking:

  - Jim and John are residents of cardiology, and they are having a sandwich in the cafeteria. John says "*I am writing* an interesting article on supraventricular tachycardia. I'll lend it to you when I've finished it." As you can see, John is not writing the article at the time of speaking. He means that he has begun to write the article but has not finished it yet. He is in the middle of writing it.

- Something that is happening for a limited period around the present (e.g., today, this week, this season, this year, etc.):

  - Our junior cardiology residents *are working* hard this term.

- Changing situations:

  - The hemodynamic condition of the patient *is getting* better.

- Temporary situations:

  - *I am living* with other residents until I can buy my own apartment.
  - *I am doing* a rotation in the CCU until the end of May.

Special use: present continuous with a future meaning.

In the following examples, doing these things is already arranged.

USES	To talk about what you have arranged to do in the near future (personal arrangements). • We *are stenting* a left main on Monday. • I *am having* dinner with an interventional cardiologist from the United States tomorrow.

We can also use the form *going to* in these sentences, but it is less natural when you talk about arrangements.

We do not use the simple present or *will* for personal arrangements.

Simple Present

The simple present tense shows an action that happens again and again (repeated action) in the present time, but not necessarily at the time of speaking.

FORM	The simple present has the following forms:
	
	• Affirmative (remember to add -*s* or -*es* to the third person singular):
	
	• Negative:
	  – I/we/you/they don't …
	  – He/she/it doesn't …
	
	• Interrogative:
	  – Do I/we/you/they …?
	  – Does he/she/it …?

Study this example: Dr. Mohd is the chairperson of the Cardiology Department. He is at an international course in Greece at this moment.

So, he *is not running* the Cardiology Department now (because he is in Greece), but *he runs* the Cardiology Department.

USES	The simple present has the following uses:
	
	• To talk about something that happens all the time or repeatedly or something that is true in general. Here, it is not important whether the action is happening at the time of speaking:
	  – I *do* interventional cardiology.
	  – Nurses *take care* of patients after an angiography procedure.
	  – For myocardial scintigraphy studies, pre-examination preparation *serves* to avoid diaphragmatic attenuation.

USES

- To say how often we do things:
  - I *begin* to make angiograms at 9.00 every morning.
  - Dr. Concha *does* angioplasty two evenings a week.
  - How often *do you go* to an international cardiology course? Once a year.

- For a permanent situation (a situation that stays the same for a long time):
  - I *work* as a cardiologist in the rehabilitation program of our hospital. I have been working there for 10 years.

- Some verbs are used only in simple tenses. These verbs are verbs of thinking or mental activity, feeling, possession, and perception, and reporting verbs. We often use *can* instead of the present tense with verbs of perception:
  - I *can understand* now why the blood pressure monitor is in such a bad condition.
  - I *can see* now the solution to the diagnostic problem or I can now see the solution to the diagnostic problem.

- The simple present is often used with adverbs of frequency such as *always, often, sometimes, rarely, never, every week*, and *twice a year*:
  - The cardiology chairperson *always* works very hard.
  - We *have* a cardiology conference *every week*.

- Simple present with a future meaning. We use it to talk about timetables, schedules, etc.:
  - What time *does* the radiation safety conference *start*? It *starts* at 9.30.

Talking about the Future

Going To

USES

- To say what we have already decided to do or what we intend to do in the future (do not use *will* in this situation):
  - I *am going* to attend the American College of Cardiology meeting next year.
  - There is a CT course in Atlanta next fall. *Are you going to* attend it?

- To say what someone has arranged to do (personal arrangements), but remember that we prefer to use the present continuous because it sounds more natural:
  - What time *are you going to meet* the vice chairperson?
  - What time *are you going to* begin the procedure?

USES

- To say what we think will happen (making predictions):
  - The patient is agitated. I think we *are not going* to get a good quality coronary scan.
  - *Oh, the patient's* chest X-ray looks terrible. "I think he is going to die soon," the cardiologist said.

- If we want to say what someone intended to do in the past but did not do, then we use *was/were going to*:
  - He *was going to* do a coronary CT on the patient but finally changed his mind and decided to do an angiogram.

- To talk about past predictions we use *was/were going to*:
  - The resident had the feeling that the patient *was going to* suffer a vagal reaction after the stress test.

Simple Future (*Will*)

FORM

The form of simple future tense:

I/We *will* or *shall* (*will* is more common than *shall*. *Shall* is often used in questions to make offers and suggestions):

- *Shall* we go to the symposium on ischemic heart disease next week? Oh! Great idea!
  You/he/she/it/they will
  Negative: *shan't, won't*

USES

- We use *will* when we decide to do something at the time of speaking (remember that in this situation, you cannot use the simple present):
  - Have you finished the report?
  - No, I haven't had time to do it.
  - OK, don't worry, I *will* do it.

- When offering, agreeing, refusing, and promising to do something, or when asking someone to do something:
  - That case looks difficult for you. Do not worry, I *will* help you out.
  - Can I have the book about mitral disease that I lent you back? Of course. I *will* give it back to you tomorrow.
  - Don't ask to perform the ultrasound examination by yourself. The consultant *won't* allow you to.
  - I promise I *will* send you a copy of the latest article on stress echocardiography as soon as I get it.
  - *Will* you help me out with this EKG, please?

You do not use *will* to say what someone has already decided to do or arranged to do (remember that in this situation we use *going to* or the present continuous).

USES

- To predict a future happening or a future situation:
  - The specialty of cardiology *will* be very different in the future.
  - Chest MRI *won't* be the same in the next two decades.

Remember that if there is something in the present situation that shows us what will happen in the future (near future), then we use *going to* instead of *will*.

USES

- With expressions such as: *probably, I am sure, I bet, I think, I suppose, I guess*:
  - I *will probably* attend the European Congress.
  - You should listen to Dr. Donald giving a conference. I am *sure* you *will* love it.
  - I *bet* the patient *will* recover satisfactorily after the IAB implantation.
  - I *guess* I *will* see you at the next annual meeting.

Future Continuous

FORM

The form is *will be* + gerund of the verb.

USES

- To say that we will be in the middle of something at a certain time in the future:
  - This time tomorrow morning I *will be performing* my first PTCA.

- To talk about things that are already planned or decided (similar to the present continuous with a future meaning):
  - We can't meet this evening. I *will be stenting the LAD* we talked about.

- To ask about people's plans, especially when we want something or want someone to do something (interrogative form):
  - *Will* you *be helping* me correct EKG reports this evening?

Future Perfect

FORM	The form is *will have* + past participle of the verb.

USES	Uses of future perfect include: • To say that something will already have happened before a certain time in the future: – I think the resident *will have arrived* by the time we begin the stress test.

Talking about the Past

Simple Past

FORM	The simple past has the following forms: • Affirmative: – The past of the regular verbs is formed by adding *-ed* to the infinitive. – The past of the irregular verbs has its own form. • Negative: – *Did/didn't* + the base form of the verb. • Questions: – *Did I/you …* + the base form of the verb

USES	Uses of the simple past tense include: • To talk about actions or situations in the past (they have already finished): – I really *enjoyed* the radiology resident's party very much. – When I *worked* as a visiting resident in Madrid, I *performed* 100 percutaneous mitral valvuloplasty procedures. • To say that one thing happened after another: – Yesterday we *had* a terrible duty. We *did* coronary angiogram in five patients, and then we *performed* a pulmonary artery thrombus extraction. • To ask or say *when* or *what* time something happened: – When *were* you on call?

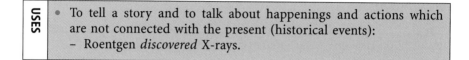

USES
- To tell a story and to talk about happenings and actions which are not connected with the present (historical events):
  - Roentgen *discovered* X-rays.

Past Continuous

FORM

The form of past continuous is *was/were* + gerund of the verb.

USES
- To say that someone was in the middle of doing something at a certain time. The action or situation had already started before this time but hadn't finished:
  - This time last year, I *was* writing the article on tricuspid valve endocarditis, which has been recently published.

Notice that the past continuous does not tell us whether an action was finished or not. Perhaps it was, perhaps it was not.

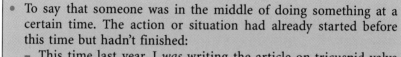

USES
- To describe a scene:
  - A lot of patients *were waiting* in the ward to have their EKGs done.

Present Perfect

FORM

The form of the present perfect tense is *have/has* + past participle of the verb.

USES
- To talk about the present result of a past action.
- To talk about a recent happening.

In the latter situation, you can use the present perfect with the following particles:

- *Just* (i.e., a short time ago); to say something has occurred a short time ago:
  - Dr. Short *has just arrived* at the hospital. He is our new pediatric cardiologist.
- *Already*; to say something has happened sooner than expected:
  - The second-year resident has *already* finished her presentation.

Remember that to talk about a recent happening we can also use the simple past:

- To talk about a period of time that continues up to the present (an unfinished period of time):
  - We use the expressions: *today, this morning, this evening, this week*, etc.
  - We often use *ever* and *never*.
- To talk about something that we are expecting. In this situation we use *yet* to show that the speaker is expecting something to happen, but only in questions and negative sentences:
  - Dr. Holms *has not arrived yet*.
- To talk about something you have never done or something you have not done during a period of time that continues up to the present:
  - I *have not reported* an EKG with a WPW syndrome since I was a resident.
- To talk about how much we have done, how many things we have done or how many times we have done something:
  - I *have punctured* that jugular vein twice.
  - Dr. Lee *has performed* 20 stress tests this week.
- To talk about situations that exists for a long time, especially if we say *always*. In this case the situation still exists now:
  - EKG *has always been* the diagnostic tool of choice in the study of supraventricular arrhythmias.
  - Dr. Sapoval *has always been* a very talented cardiologist.

We also use the present perfect with these expressions:

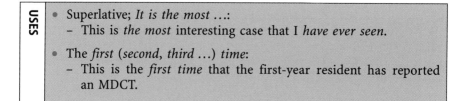

USES

- Superlative; *It is the most ...*:
  - This is *the most* interesting case that I *have ever seen*.
- The *first (second, third ...) time*:
  - This is the *first time* that the first-year resident has reported an MDCT.

Present Perfect Continuous

This tense shows an action that began in the past and has gone on up to the present time.

FORM

Its form is *have/has* been + gerund.

USES

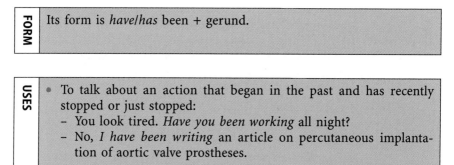

- To talk about an action that began in the past and has recently stopped or just stopped:
  - You look tired. *Have you been working* all night?
  - No, *I have been writing* an article on percutaneous implantation of aortic valve prostheses.
- To ask or say how long something has been happening. In this case the action or situation began in the past and is still happening or has just stopped.
  - Dr. Rubens and Dr. Palazuelos *have been working* together *from* the beginning of this project.

We use the following particles:

USES

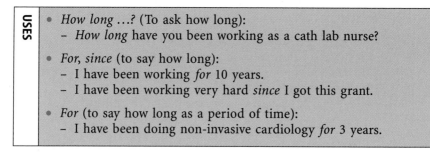

- *How long ...?* (To ask how long):
  - *How long* have you been working as a cath lab nurse?
- *For, since* (to say how long):
  - I have been working *for* 10 years.
  - I have been working very hard *since* I got this grant.
- *For* (to say how long as a period of time):
  - I have been doing non-invasive cardiology *for* 3 years.

Do not use *for* in expressions with *all*: "I have been working as a cardiologist all my life" (not "*for all* my life").

USES	• *Since* (to say the beginning of a period): – I have been teaching cardiac ultrasound *since* 1994.

In the present perfect continuous tense, the important thing is the action itself, and it does not matter whether the action is finished or not. The action can be finished (just finished) or not (still happening).

In the present perfect, the important thing is the result of the action and not the action itself. The action is completely finished.

Past Perfect

The past perfect tense shows an action that happened in the past before another past action. It is the past of the present perfect.

FORM	Its form is *had* + past participle of the verb.

USES	• To say that something had already happened before something else happened: – When I arrived at the cath lab, the interventional cardiologist *had* already *begun* the rotablator atherectomy procedure.

Past Perfect Continuous

This tense shows an action that began in the past and went on up to a time in the past. It is the past of the present perfect continuous.

FORM	Its form is *had been* + gerund of the verb.

USES	• To say how long something had been happening before something else happened: – She *had been working* as a pediatric cardiologist for 40 years before she was awarded the Amplatz prize.

Subjunctive

Imagine this situation:

- The cardiac surgeon says to the interventional cardiologist, "Why don't you do a PTCA on the patient with left main disease?"

The surgeon proposes (that) the cardiologist do a PTCA procedure on the patient with left main *coronary* disease.

The subjunctive is formed always with the base form of the verb (the infinitive without *to*):

- I suggest (that) you *work* harder.
- She recommended (that) he *give up* smoking while working.
- He insisted (that) she *perform an ultrasound examination* on the patient as soon as possible.
- He demanded (that) the nurse *treat him* more politely.

Note that the subjunctive of the verb *to be* is usually passive:

- He insisted (that) the EKG *be evaluated* immediately.
  You can use the subjunctive after:
- Propose
- Suggest
- Recommend
- Insist
- Demand

You can use the subjunctive for the past, present or future:

- He *suggested* (that) the resident *change* the treatment.
- He *recommends* (that) his patients *give up* smoking.

Should is sometimes used instead of the subjunctive:

- The doctor recommended that *I should give up smoking*.

Wish, If Only, Would

Wish

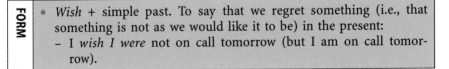

FORM	• *Wish* + simple past. To say that we regret something (i.e., that something is not as we would like it to be) in the present: – I *wish I were* not on call tomorrow (but I am on call tomorrow).

<table>
<tr><td>FORM</td><td>

- *Wish* + past perfect. To say that we regret something that happened or did not happen in the past:
  - *I wish he hadn't treated* the patient's family so badly (but he treated the patient's family badly).

- *Wish* + *would* + infinitive without *to* when we want something to happen or change or somebody to do something:
  - *I wish you wouldn't walk* so slowly (note that the speaker is complaining about the present situation or the way people do things).

</td></tr>
</table>

If Only

If only can be used in exactly the same way as *wish*. It has the same meaning as *wish* but is more dramatic:

<table>
<tr><td>FORM</td><td>

- *If only* + past simple (expresses regret in the present):
  - *If only I were not* on call tomorrow.

- *If only* + past perfect (expresses regret in the past):
  - *If only he hadn't treated* the patient's family so badly.

</td></tr>
</table>

After *wish* and *if only* we use *were* (with *I*, *he*, *she*, *it*) instead of *was*, and we do not normally use *would*, although sometimes it is possible, or *would have*.

When referring to the present or future, *wish* and *if only* are followed by a past tense, and when referring to the past by a past perfect tense.

Would

Would is used:

<table>
<tr><td>USES</td><td>

- As a modal verb in offers, invitations and requests (i.e., to ask someone to do something):
  - *Would* you help me write an article on heart tumors? (Request)
  - *Would* you like to come to the residents' party tonight? (Offer and invitation)

- After *wish* (see "*Wish*")

- In *if* sentences (see "Conditionals")

- Sometimes as the past of *will* (in reported speech):
  - Dr. Ho: "I will do your stress test next week."
  - Patient: "The doctor said that he *would* do my stress test next week."

</td></tr>
</table>

USES

- When you remember things that often happened (similar to *used to*):
  - When we were residents, we used to prepare the clinical cases together.
  - When we were residents, we *would* prepare the clinical cases together.

Modal Verbs

FORM

- A modal verb has always the same form.
- There is no -*s* ending in the third person singular, no -*ing* form, and no -*ed* form.
- After a modal verb we use the infinitive without *to* (i.e., the base form of the verb).

These are the English modal verbs:

- *Can* (past form is *could*)
- *Could* (also a modal with its own meaning)
- *May* (past form is *might*)
- *Might* (also a modal with its own meaning)
- *Will*
- *Would*
- *Shall*
- *Should*
- *Ought to*
- *Must*
- *Need*
- *Dare*

We use modal verbs to talk about:

- Ability
- Necessity
- Possibility
- Certainty
- Permission
- Obligation

Expressing Ability

To express ability we can use:

- *Can* (only in the present tense).
- *Could* (only in the past tense).
- *Be able to* (in all tenses).

Ability in the Present

Can (more usual) or *am/is/are able to* (less usual):

- Dr. Williams *can* treat extremely difficult left main coronary artery stenoses.
- Dr. Douglas *is able to* dilate pulmonary valve stenoses in children.
- *Can* you speak medical English? Yes, I *can.*
- *Are you able to* speak medical English? Yes, I *am.*

Ability in the Past

The forms are *could* (past form of *can*) or *was/were able to*:

<table>
<tr>
<td>USES</td>
<td>

- We use *could* to say to say that someone had the *general* ability to do something:
  - When I was a resident, I *could* speak German.

- We use *was/were able to* say that someone managed to do something in one particular situation (*specific* ability to do something):
  - When I was a resident, I *was able to* do 15 duties in 1 month.

- *Managed to* can replace *was able to*:
  - When I was a resident, I *managed to* do 15 duties in 1 month.

- We use *could have* to say that we had the ability to do something but we did not do it:
  - He *could have* been a surgeon but he became a cardiologist instead.

- Sometimes we use *could* to talk about ability in a situation which we are imagining (here *could = would be able to*):
  - I *couldn't* do your job; I'm not clever enough.

- We use *will be able to* talk about ability with a future meaning:
  - If you keep on studying cardiological English, then you *will be able to* write scientific articles very soon.

</td>
</tr>
</table>

Expressing Necessity

Necessity means that you cannot avoid doing something.
To say that it is necessary to do something we can use *must* or *have to*.

- Necessity in the present: *must, have/has to*.
- Necessity in the past: *had to*.
- Necessity in the future: *must* or *will have to*.
- Notice that to express necessity in the past we do not use *must*.

There are some differences between *must* and *have to*:

<table>
<tr><td>USES</td><td>

- We use *must* when the speaker is expressing personal feelings or authority, saying what he or she thinks is necessary:
  - Your chest X-ray film shows severe emphysema. You *must* give up smoking.

- We use *have to* when the speaker is not expressing personal feelings or authority. The speaker is just giving facts or expressing the authority of another person (external authority), often a law or a rule:
  - All cardiology residents *have to* learn how to evaluate an EKG in their first year of residency.

- If we want to express that there is necessity to avoid doing something, then we use *mustn't* (i.e., *not allowed to*):
  - You *mustn't* eat anything before the angiogram.

</td></tr>
</table>

Expressing No Necessity

To express that there is no necessity we can use the negative forms of *need* or *have* to:

- No necessity in the present: *needn't* or *don't/doesn't have to*.
- No necessity in the past: *didn't need, didn't have to*.
- No necessity in the future: *won't have to*.

Notice that "there is no necessity to do something" is completely different from "there is a necessity not to do something."
In conclusion, we use *mustn't* when we are not allowed to do something or when there is a necessity not to do it, and we use the negative form of *have to* or *needn't* when there is no necessity to do something but we can do it if we want to:

- The cardiologist says *I mustn't* get overtired before the procedure but *I needn't* stay in bed.

- The cardiologist says *I mustn't* get overtired before the procedure but *I don't have to* stay in bed.

Expressing Possibility

To express possibility we can use *can, could, may,* or *might* (from more to less certainty: can, may, might, could).

But also note that *can* is used of ability (or capacity) to do something; *may,* with permission or sanction to do it.

Possibility in the Present

To say that something is possible we use *can, may, might, could*:

- High doses of digoxin *can* cause partial blindness (high level of certainty)
- Digoxin *may* cause partial blindness (moderate to high level of certainty).
- Digoxin *might* cause nausea and vomiting (moderate to low level of certainty).
- Digoxin *could* cause renal failure.

Possibility in the Past

USES

- To say something was possible in the past we use *may have, might have, could have*:
  - The lesion *might have* been detected on ultrasound.

- *Could have* is also used to say that something was a possibility or opportunity but it didn't happen:
  - You were lucky to be treated with primary angioplasty and stenting, otherwise you *could have* died.

- I *couldn't have* done something (i.e., I wouldn't have been able to do it if I had wanted or tried to do it):
  - She *couldn't have* heard that systolic murmur because it was extremely mild.

Possibility in the Future

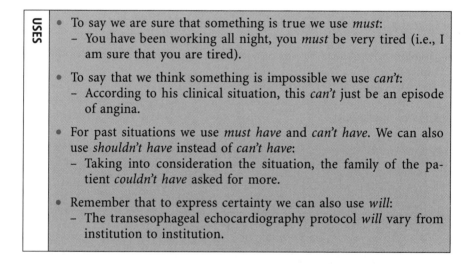

USES

- To talk about possible future actions or happenings we use *may*, *might*, *could* (especially in suggestions):
  - I don't know where to do my last six months of residency. I *may/might* go to the States.
  - We *could* meet later in the hospital to write the article, couldn't we?

- When we are talking about possible future plans we can also use the continuous form *may/might/could be + -ing* form:
  - I *could be going* to the next AHA meeting.

Expressing Certainty

USES

- To say we are sure that something is true we use *must*:
  - You have been working all night, you *must* be very tired (i.e., I am sure that you are tired).

- To say that we think something is impossible we use *can't*:
  - According to his clinical situation, this *can't* just be an episode of angina.

- For past situations we use *must have* and *can't have*. We can also use *shouldn't have* instead of *can't have*:
  - Taking into consideration the situation, the family of the patient *couldn't have* asked for more.

- Remember that to express certainty we can also use *will*:
  - The transesophageal echocardiography protocol *will* vary from institution to institution.

Expressing Permission

To talk about permission we can use *can*, *may* (more formal than *can*), or *be allowed to.*

Permission in the Present

Can, may, or *am/is/are allowed to*:

- You *can* smoke if you like.
- You *are allowed to* smoke.
- You *may* attend the congress.

Permission in the Past

Was/were allowed to:

- *Were you allowed to* go into the cath lab without surgical scrubs?

Permission in the Future

- *Will be allowed to*:
  - I *will be allowed to* leave the hospital when my duty is finished.

- To ask for permission we use *can, may, could,* or *might* (from less to more formal) but not *be allowed to*:
  - Hi Hannah, *can* I borrow your digital camera? (If you are asking for a friend's digital camera)
  - Dr. Chang, *may* I borrow your digital camera? (If you are talking to an acquaintance)
  - *Could* I use your digital camera, Dr. Coltrane? (If you are talking to a colleague you do not know at all)
  - *Might* I use your digital camera, Dr. Escaned? (If you are asking for the chairperson's digital camera)

Expressing Obligation or Giving Advice

Obligation means that something is the proper thing to do. When we want to say what we think is a good thing to do or the right thing to do we use *should* or *ought to* (a little stronger than *should*).

Should and *ought to* can be used for giving advice:

- You *ought* to sleep.
- You *should* work out.
- You *ought to* give up smoking.
- *Should* he see a doctor? Yes, I think he *should*.

Conditionals

Conditional sentences have two parts:

1. "If" clause.
2. Main clause.

In the sentence "If I were you, then I would go to the annual meeting of cardiology residents," *if I were you* is the if clause, and *then I would go to the annual meeting of cardiology residents* is the main clause.

The if clause can come before or after the main clause. We often put a comma when the if clause comes first.

Main Types of Conditional Sentences

Type 0

This type is used to talk about things that always are true (general truths).

If + simple present + simple present:

- *If* you inject agitated saline, then the left atrium becomes apparent.
- *If* you see free air in the chest, then the patient has a pneumothorax.
- *If* you drink too much alcohol, then you get a sore head.
- *If* you take drugs habitually, then you become addicted.

Note that the examples above refer to things that are normally true. They make no reference to the future; they represent a present simple concept. This is the basic (or classic) form of the conditional type 0.

There are possible variations of this form. In the if clause and in the main clause, we can use the present continuous, present perfect simple or present perfect continuous instead of the present simple. In the main clause, we can also use the imperative instead of the present simple:

- Residents only get certificate *if* they *have attended* the course regularly.
  So the type 0 form can be reduced to:
- *If* + present form + present form or imperative.

Present forms include the present simple, present continuous, present perfect simple, and present perfect continuous.

Type 1

This type is used to talk about future situations that the speaker thinks are likely to happen (the speaker is thinking about a real possibility in the future).

If + simple present + future simple (*will*):

- *If* I find something new about the percutaneous treatment of aortic stenosis, then I will tell you.
- *If* we analyze antiarrhythmic agents, then we will be able to infer principles about their effect over systolic function.

These examples refer to future things that are possible and it is quite probable that they will happen. This is the basic (or classic) form of the conditional type 1.

There are possible variations of the basic form. In the if clause, we can use the present continuous, the present perfect or the present perfect continuous instead of the present simple. In the main clause, we can use the future continuous, future perfect simple or future perfect continuous instead of the future simple. Modals such as *can*, *may*, or *might* are also possible.

So, the form of type 1 can be reduced to *if* + present form + future form.

Future forms include the future simple, future continuous, future perfect simple, and future perfect continuous.

Type 2

Type 2 is used to talk about future situations that the speaker thinks are possible but not probable (the speaker is imagining a possible future situation) or to talk about unreal situations in the present.

If + simple past + conditional (*would*):

- Peter, *if* you *studied* harder, then you *would* be better prepared for doing your CAQ in echocardiography. (This sentence tells us that Peter is not supposed to be studying hard.)
- *If* I *were* you, then I *would* go to the Annual Meeting of Interventional Cardiology. (But I am not you.).
- *If* I *were* a resident *again*, then I *would* go to Harvard Medical School for a whole year to complete my training period. (But I am not a resident.)

There are possible variations of the basic form. In the if clause, we can use the past continuous instead of the past simple. In the main clause, we can use *could* or *might* instead of *would*.

So, the form of type 2 can be reduced to *if* + past simple or continuous + *would*, *could* or *might*.

Type 3

Type 3 is used to talk about past situations that did not happen (impossible actions in the past).

If + past perfect + perfect conditional (*would have*):

- *If* I *had known* the patient's symptoms, then I *would have* not missed the ST-segment elevation on the EKG.

As you can see, we are talking about the past. The real situation is that I did not know the patient's symptoms, so that I did not notice the small ST-segment elevation.

This is the basic or classic form of the third type of conditional. There are possible variations. In the if clause, we can use the past perfect continuous instead of the past perfect simple. In the main clause, we can use the continuous form of the perfect conditional instead of the perfect conditional simple. *Would probably*, *could*, or *might* instead of *would* are also possible (when we are not sure about something).

In Case

"The interventional cardiologist wears two pairs of latex gloves *in case* one of them tears." *In case one of them tears*, because it is possible that one of them tears during the intervention (in the future).

Note that we do not use *will* after *in case*. We use a present tense after *in case* when we are talking about the future.

In case is not the same as *if*. Compare these sentences:

1. We'll buy some more food and drink *if* the new residents come to our department's party. (Perhaps the new residents will come to our party. If they come, we will buy some more food and drink; if they don't come, we won't.)
2. We will buy some food and drink *in case* the new residents come to our department's party. (Perhaps the new residents will come to our department's party. We will buy some more food and drink whether they come or not.)

We can also use *in case* to say why someone did something in the past:

- He rang the bell again *in case* the nurse hadn't heard it the first time. (Because it was possible that the nurse hadn't heard it the first time.)

In case of (= if there is):

- *In case of* pregnancy, don't do an X-ray examination.

Unless

- "Don't take these pills *unless* you are extremely anxious." (Don't take these pills except if you are extremely anxious.) This sentence means that you can take the pills only if you are extremely anxious.

We use *unless* to make an exception to something we say.

We often use *unless* in warnings:

- *Unless* you submit the article today, it won't be accepted for publication in *Circulation*.

It is also possible to use *if* in a negative sentence instead of *unless*:

- Don't take those pills *if you aren't* extremely anxious.
- *If you don't submit* the article today, it won't be accepted for publication in *Circulation*.

As Long As, Provided (That), Providing (That)

These expressions mean *but only if*:

- You can use my new pen to sign your report *as long as* you write carefully (i.e., *but only if* you write carefully).
- Going by car to the hospital is convenient *provided* (*that*) you have somewhere to park (i.e., *but only if* you have somewhere to park).
- *Providing* (*that*) she studies the clinical cases, she will deliver a bright presentation.

Passive Voice

Study these examples:

1. The first ultrasound examination was performed at our hospital in 1980 (passive sentence).
2. Someone performed the first ultrasound examination at our hospital in 1980 (active sentence).

Both sentences are correct and mean the same. They are two different ways of saying the same thing, but in the passive sentence, we try to make the object of the active sentence ("the first ultrasound examination") more important by putting it at the beginning. Therefore, we prefer to use the passive when it is not that important who or what did the action. In the example above, it is not so important (or not known) who performed the first ultrasound examination.

Active sentence:
- Fleming (subject) discovered (active verb) penicillin (object) in 1950.

Passive sentence:
- Penicillin (subject) was discovered (passive verb) by Fleming (agent) in 1950.

The passive verb is formed by putting the verb *to be* into the same tense as the active verb and adding the past participle of the active verb:

- Discovered (active verb) – was discovered (*be* + past participle of the active verb).

The object (*penicillin*) of an active verb becomes the subject of the passive verb. The subject (*Fleming*) of an active verb becomes the agent of the passive verb. We can leave out the agent if it is not important to mention it or we do not know it. If we want to mention it, we will put it at the end of the sentence preceded by the particle *by* (" ... Fleming").

Some sentences have two objects, indirect and direct. In these sentences, the passive subject can be either the direct object or the indirect object of the active sentence:

- The doctor gave the patient a new treatment.

There are two possibilities:

- A new treatment was given to the patient.
- The patient was given a new treatment.

Passive Forms of Present and Past Tenses

Simple Present

Active:
- Cardiologists review the most interesting patients in the clinical session every day.

Passive:
- The most interesting patients are reviewed in the clinical session every day.

Simple Past

Active:
- The nurse checked the renal function of the patient before the procedure.

Passive:
- The renal function of the patient was checked before the procedure.

Present Continuous

Active:
- Dr. Goodyear is performing an angiogram right now.

Passive:
- An angiogram is being performed right now.

Past Continuous

Active:
- They were carrying the patient to the ICU.

Passive:
- The patient was being carried to the ICU.

Present Perfect

Active:
- The cardiologist has performed ten TEEs this morning.

Passive:
- Ten TEEs have been performed this morning.

Past Perfect

Active:
- They had sent the angiogram's films before the operation started.

Passive:
- The angiogram's films had been sent before the operation started.

In sentences of the type "people say/consider/know/think/believe/expect/understand ... that ...," such as "Doctors consider that AIDS is a fatal disease," we have two possible passive forms:

1. AIDS is considered a fatal disease.
2. It is considered that AIDS is a fatal disease.

Have/Get Something Done

> **FORM**
>
> The form is *have/get* + object + past participle.

USES
- Get is a little more informal than *have*, and it is often used in informal spoken English:
  - You should *get* your ultrasound machine tested.
  - You should *have* your ultrasound machine tested.

When we want to say that we do not want to do something ourselves, and we arrange for someone to do it for us, we use the expression *have something done*:

- The patient had all his metal objects removed in order to prevent accidents during the MR examination.
  Sometimes the expression *have something done* has a different meaning:
- John had his tooth broken playing a paddle match. He needed the antibiotics protocol for endocarditis prevention because he has a significant mitral regurgitation.

It is obvious that this does not mean that he arranged for somebody to break his tooth. With this meaning, we use *have something done* to say that something (often something not nice) happened to someone.

Supposed To

Supposed to can be used in the following ways:

It can be used like *said* to:

- The chairperson is *supposed to* be the one who runs the department.

To say what is planned or arranged (and this is often different from what really happens):

- The fourth-year resident is *supposed to* do this angiogram.

To say what is not allowed or not advisable:

- She was not *supposed to* be on call yesterday.

Reported Speech

Imagine that you want to tell someone else what the patient said. You can either repeat the patient's words or use reported speech.
  The reporting verb (*said* in the examples below) can come before or after the reported clause, but it usually comes before the reported clause. When the reporting verb comes before, we can use *that* to introduce the reported clause or we can leave it out (leaving it out is more informal).

The reporting verb can report statements and thoughts, questions, orders, and requests.

Reporting in the Present

When the reporting verb is in the present tense, it is not necessary to change the tense of the verb:

- "I'll help you guys with this patient," he says.
- He says (that) he will help us explore this patient.
- "The mitral valvuloplasty will take place this morning," he says.
- He says (that) the valvuloplasty will take place this morning.

Reporting in the Past

When the reporting verb is in the past tense, the verb in direct speech usually changes in the following ways:

- Simple present changes to simple past.
- Present continuous changes to past continuous.
- Simple past changes to past perfect.
- Past continuous changes to past perfect continuous.
- Present perfect changes to past perfect.
- Present perfect continuous changes to past perfect continuous.
- Past perfect says the same.
- Future changes to conditional.
- Future continuous changes to conditional continuous.
- Future perfect changes to conditional perfect.
- Conditional stays the same.
- Present forms of modal verbs stay the same.
- Past forms of modal verbs stay the same.

Pronouns, adjectives and adverbs also change. Here are some examples:

- First person singular changes to third person singular.
- Second person singular changes to first person singular.
- First person plural changes to third person plural.
- Second person plural changes to first person plural.
- Third person singular changes to third person plural.
- *Now* changes to *then*.
- *Today* changes to *that day*.
- *Tomorrow* changes to *the day after*.
- *Yesterday* changes to *the day before*.
- *This* changes to *that*.
- *Here* changes *to there*.
- *Ago* changes *to before*.

It is not always necessary to change the verb when you use reported speech. If you are reporting something and you feel that it is still true, then you do not need to change the tense of the verb, but if you want, you can do it:

- The treatment of choice for severe urticaria after intracoronary contrast injection is epinephrine.
- He said (that) the treatment of choice for severe urticaria after intracoronary contrast administration is epinephrine.

Or

- He said (that) the treatment of choice for severe urticaria after intracoronary contrast administration was epinephrine.

Reporting Questions

Yes/No Questions

We use *whether* or *if*:

- Do you smoke?
  - The doctor asked if I smoked.
- Have you had any urticaria after iodine contrast administration?
  - The doctor asked me whether I had had any urticaria after iodine contrast administration.
- Are you taking any pills or medicines at the moment?
  - The doctor asked me if I was taking any pills or medicines at that moment.

Wh... Questions

We use the same question word as in the *wh...* question:

- W*hat* do you mean by saying, you are "feeling under the weather?"
  - The doctor asked me what I meant by saying "I was feeling under the weather."
- W*hy* do you think you "feel under the weather?"
  - The doctor asked me why I thought I felt "under the weather."
- W*hen* do you "feel under the weather?"
  - The doctor asked me when I felt "under the weather."
- *How often* do you have headaches?
  - The doctor asked me how often I had headaches.

Reported Questions

Reported questions have the following characteristics:

- The word order is different from that of the original question. The verb follows the subject as in an ordinary statement.
- The auxiliary verb *do* is not used.
- There is no question mark.
- The verb changes in the same way as in direct speech.

Study the following examples:

- How old are you?
  - The doctor asked me how old I was.
- Do you smoke?
  - The doctor asked me if I smoked.

Reporting Orders and Requests

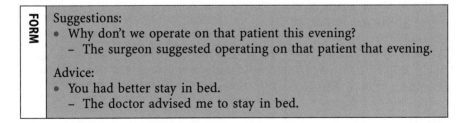

FORM	*Tell* (pronoun) + object (indirect) + infinitive:
	• Take the pills before meals.
	– The doctor *told* me to take the pills before meals.
	• You mustn't smoke.
	– The doctor *told* me not to smoke.

Reporting Suggestions and Advice

Suggestions and advice are reported in the following forms:

FORM	Suggestions:
	• Why don't we operate on that patient this evening?
	– The surgeon suggested operating on that patient that evening.
	Advice:
	• You had better stay in bed.
	– The doctor advised me to stay in bed.

Questions

In sentences with *to be*, *to have* (in its auxiliary form), and modal verbs, we usually make questions by changing the word order:

> **FORM**
>
> Affirmative:
> - *You are* a cardiologist.
>   - Interrogative: *Are you* a cardiologist?
>
> Negative:
> - *You are not* a cardiologist.
>   - Interrogative: *Aren't you* a cardiologist?

In simple present questions, we use *do/does*:

- His stomach hurts after having the loading dose of clopidogrel.
- *Does* his stomach hurt after having the loading dose of clopidogrel?

In simple past questions we use *did*:

- The nurse arrived on time.
- *Did* the nurse arrive on time?

If *who/what/which* is the subject of the sentence, then we do not use *do*:

- Someone paged Dr. Yu.
- *Who* paged Dr. Yu?

If *who/what/which* is the object of the sentence we use *did*:

- Dr. Yu paged someone.
- *Whom* did Dr. Yu page?

When we ask somebody and begin the question with *Do you know ...?* or *Could you tell me ...?*, the rest of the question maintains the affirmative sentence's word order:

- Where is the reading room?
But
- Do you know where the reading room is?
- Where is the library?
But
- Could you tell me where the library is?

Reported questions also maintain the affirmative sentence's word order:

- Dr. Wilson asked "How are you?"

But

- Dr. Wilson asked me how I was.

Short answers are possible in questions where *be, do, can, have,* and *might* are auxiliary verbs:

- *Do* you smoke?
  – Yes, I *do.*
- *Did* you smoke?
  – No, I *didn't.*
- *Can* you walk?
  – Yes, I *can.*

We also use auxiliary verbs with *so* (affirmative) and *neither* or *nor* (negative) changing the word order:

- I am feeling tired.
  – *So* am I.
- I can't remember the name of the disease.
  – *Neither* can I.
- Is he going to pass the boards?
  – I think *so.*
- Will you be on call tomorrow?
  – I guess *not.*
- Will you be off call the day after tomorrow?
  – I hope *so.*
- Has the chairperson been invited to the party?
  – I'm afraid *so.*

Tag Questions

We use a positive tag question with a negative sentence and vice versa:

- The first-year resident isn't feeling very well today, is he?
- You are working late at the lab, aren't you?

After *let's,* the tag question is *shall we?*

- Let's read a couple of articles, *shall we?*

After the imperative, the tag question is *will you?*

- Turn of the viewer, *will you?*

Infinitive/-*ing*

Verb + -*ing*

There are certain verbs that are usually used in the structure verb + -*ing* when followed by another verb:

- *Stop*: Please *stop talking*.
- *Finish*: *I've finished translating* the article into English.
- *Enjoy*: *I enjoy talking* to patients.
- *Mind*: I *don't mind being* told what to do.
- *Suggest*: Dr. Svenson *suggested going* to the ER and trying to evacuate the pericardial effusion that was found in that patient.
- *Dislike*: She *dislikes going* out late after a night on call.
- *Imagine*: *I can't imagine you performing* a PTCA procedure. You told me you hate blood and working under pressure.
- *Regret*: He *regrets having gone* 2 minutes before his patient had seizures.
- *Admit*: The resident *admitted forgetting* to order digoxin for Mrs. Smith.
- *Consider*: Have you *considered finishing* your residence in the United States?
- Other verbs that follow this structure are: *avoid, deny, involve, practice, miss, postpone,* and *risk.*

The following expressions also take -*ing*:

- *Give up*: Are you trying to *give up smoking?*
- *Keep on*: She *kept on interrupting* me while I was speaking.
- *Go on*: *Go on studying*, the exam will be next month.

When we are talking about finished actions, we can also use the verb *to have*:

- The resident *admitted forgetting* to write Mrs. Smith's discharge report.
- The resident *admitted having forgotten* to write down Mrs. Smith's discharge report.

And, with some of these verbs (*admit, deny, regret,* and *suggest*), you also can use a "that ..." structure:

- The resident *admitted forgetting* to write Mrs. Smith's discharge report.
- The resident *admitted that he had forgotten* to write Mrs. Smith's discharge report.

Verb + Infinitive

When followed by another verb, these verbs are used with verb + infinitive structure:

- Agree: The patient *agreed to give up* smoking.
- Refuse: The patient *refused to give up* smoking.
- Promise: I *promised to give up* smoking.
- Threaten: Dr. Font *threatened to close* the cardiology department.
- Offer: The unions *offered to negotiate*.
- Decide: Dr. Knight's patients *decided to leave* the waiting room.

Other verbs that follow this structure are *attempt, manage, fail, plan, arrange, afford, forget, learn, dare, end, appear, seem, pretend, need,* and *intend*.

There are two possible structures after these verbs: *want, ask, expect, help, would like,* and *would prefer*:

- Verb + infinitive: I *asked to see* Dr. Knight, the surgeon who operated on my patient.
- Verb + object + infinitive: I *asked Dr. Knight to inform* me about my patient.

There is only one possible structure after the following verbs: *tell, order, remind, warn, force, invite, enable, teach, persuade,* and *get*:

- Verb + object + infinitive: *Remind me to talk* to the patient's family tomorrow before 10 a.m.

There are two possible structures after the following verbs:

- *Advise*:
    - I *wouldn't advise learning* at that old hospital.
    - I *wouldn't advise you to learn* at that old hospital.
- *Allow*:
    - They *don't allow smoking* in the CT room.
    - They *don't allow you to smoke* in the CT room.
- *Permit*:
    - They *don't permit eating* in the residents reading room.
    - They *don't permit you to eat* in the residents reading room.

When you use *make* and *let*, you should use the structure: verb + base form (instead of verb + infinitive):

- Blood *makes me feel* dizzy (you cannot say: Blood *makes me to feel* ...)
- Dr. Concha *wouldn't let me repeat* the angiogram.

After the following expressions and verbs, you can use either *-ing* or the infinitive: *like, hate, love, can't stand,* and *can't bear*:

- She *can't stand being* alone while she is performing an ultrasound examination.
- She *can't stand to be* alone while she is performing an ultrasound examination.

After the following verbs, you can use *-ing* but not the infinitive: *dislike, enjoy,* and *mind*:

- I *enjoy being* alone. (*Not* "I *enjoy to be alone*")

Would like, a polite way of saying *I want,* is followed by the infinitive:

- *Would you like to be* the chairperson of the non-invasive division of the department?

Begin, start, and *continue* can be followed by either *-ing* or the infinitive:
- The patient *began to improve* after the administration of diuretics.
- The patient *began improving* after the administration of diuretics.

With some verbs, such as *remember* and *try,* the use of *-ing* and infinitive after them have different meanings:

Remember:
- *I did not remember to place* the tip of the catheter far enough from the AV node. (I forgot to place the catheter properly.)
- *I could remember (myself) placing* the tip of a catheter far enough from the AV node that day. (I can recall how I placed the catheter.)
Try:
- The patient *tried to keep* her eyes open.
- If your headache persists, *try asking for* a change on your medication.

Verb + Preposition + *-ing*

If a verb comes after a preposition, that verb ends in *-ing*:

- Are you interested *in working* for our hospital?
- What are the advantages *of developing* new interventional techniques?
- She's not very good *at learning* languages.

You can use *-ing* with before and after:
- Discharge Mr. Brown *before operating* on the aneurism.
- What did you do *after finishing* your residence?

You can use *by + -ing* to explain how something happened:
- You can improve your medical English *by reading* scientific articles.

You can use *-ing* after *without*:

- Jim got to the hospital, *without realizing* he had his locker keys at home.

Be careful with *to*, because it can either be a part of the infinitive or a preposition:

- I'm looking forward *to see* you again (this is *not* correct).
- I'm looking forward *to seeing* you again.
- I'm looking forward *to the next European congress*.

Review the following verb + preposition expressions:

- *Succeed in* finding a job.
- *Feel like* going out tonight?
- *Think about* operating on that patient.
- *Dream of* being a cardiologist.
- *Disapprove of* smoking.
- *Look forward to* hearing from you.
- *Insist on* inviting me to chair the session.
- *Apologize for* keeping Dr. Chang waiting.
- *Accuse (someone) of* telling lies.
- *Suspected of* having AIDS.
- *Stop from* leaving the ward.
- *Thank (someone) for* being helpful.
- *Forgive (someone) for* not writing to me.
- *Warn (someone) against* carrying on smoking.

The following are some examples of expressions + *-ing*:

- I don't feel *like going out* tonight.
- It's no use *trying to persuade* her.
- There's no point *in waiting for* him.
- It's not worth taking a taxi. The hospital *is only a short walk from* here.
- It's worth *looking again at* that radiograph.
- I am having difficulty *trying to cross* the stenosis.
- I am having trouble *trying to cross* the stenosis.

Countable and Uncountable Nouns

Countable Nouns

Countable nouns are things we can count. We can make them plural.

Before singular countable nouns you may use *a/an*:

- You will be attended to by *a* cardiologist.
- Dr. Barba is looking for *an* invasive cardiologist.

Remember to use *a/an* for jobs:

- I'm *a* cardiologist.
  Before plural countable nouns you use *some* as a general rule:
- I've read *some* good articles on coronary CT lately.
  Do not use *some* when you are talking about general things:
- Generally speaking, I like cardiology books.
  You have to use *some* when you mean *some, but not all*:
- Some doctors carry a stethoscope.

Uncountable Nouns

Uncountable nouns are things we cannot count. They have no plural.
    You cannot use *a/an* before an uncountable noun; in this case you have
to use *the, some, any, much, this, his*, etc., ... or leave the uncountable
noun alone, without the article:

- The chairperson gave me *an* advice. (*Not* correct)
- The chairperson gave me *some* advice (or a piece of advice).

Many nouns can be used as countable or uncountable nouns. Usually there
is a difference in their meaning.

- I had many experiences on my rotation at the *children's hospital* (countable).
- I need experience to become a good *cardiologist* (uncountable).

Some nouns are uncountable in English but often countable in other
languages: *advice, baggage, behavior, bread, chaos, furniture, information,
luggage, news, permission, progress, scenery, traffic, travel, trouble,* and
weather.

Articles: *A/An* and *The*

The speaker uses *a/an* when it is the first time he/she talks about something, but once the listener knows what the speaker is talking about, he/she uses *the*:

- I did *an* ultrasound and a chest plain film. The ultrasound was completely normal.

We use *the* when it is clear which thing or person we mean:

- Can you turn off *the* light?
- Where is *the* Non-Invasive Cardiology Division, please?

As a general rule, we say:

- The police
- The bank
- The post office ("Post Office," in British English)
- The fire department
- The doctor
- The hospital
- The dentist

We say *the sea, the sky, the ground, the city,* and *the country.*

We don't use *the* with the names of meals:

- What did you have for lunch/breakfast/dinner?

But we use *a* when there is an adjective before a noun:

- Thank you. It was *a* delicious dinner.

We use *the* for musical instruments:

- Can you play *the* piano?

We use *the* with absolute adjectives (adjectives used as nouns). The meaning is always plural. For example:

- The rich
- The old
- The blind
- The sick
- The disabled
- The injured
- The poor

- The young
- The deaf
- The dead
- The unemployed
- The homeless.

We use *the* with nationality words (note that nationality words always begin with a capital letter):

- *The* British, *the* Dutch, *the* Spanish.

We do not use *the* before a noun when we mean something in general:

- I love doctors (not *the* doctors).

With the words *school, college, prison, jail,* and *church,* we use *the* when we mean *the buildings* and leave the substantives alone otherwise. We say *go to bed, go to work,* and *go home.* We do not use *the* in these cases.

We use *the* with geographical names according to the following rules:

- References to continents do not use *the*:
  – Our new resident comes from Asia.
- References to countries/states do not use *the*:
  – The patient that underwent a cath this morning came from Gibraltar.
  (Except for country names that include words such as Republic, Kingdom, and States ..., e.g., *the* United States of America, *the* United Kingdom, and *The* Netherlands).

- As a general rule, references to cities do not use *the*:
  – The next cardiology congress will be held in Barcelona.
- References to islands don't use *the* with individual islands but do use it with groups:
  – Dr. Leon comes from Sicily and her husband from *the* Canary Islands.
- References to lakes do not use *the*; oceans, seas, rivers and canals do use it:
  – Lake Windermere is beautiful.
  – The Panama Canal links the Atlantic Ocean to the Pacific Ocean.

We use *the* with buildings, universities, etc., according to the following rules:

- Streets, roads, avenues, boulevards and squares do not take *the*:
  – The hospital is sited at 15th Avenue.
- Airports don't take *the*:
  – The plane arrived at JFK airport.
- We use *the* before publicly recognized buildings: *the* White House, *the* Empire State Building, *the* Louvre Museum, *the* Prado Museum.

- We use *the* before names with of: *the* Tower of London, *the* Great Wall of China.
- Universities don't take *the*: I studied at Harvard.

Word Order

The order of adjectives is discussed in the section "Adjectives" under the heading "Adjective Order."

The verb and the object of the verb normally go together:

- I *studied cardiology* because I like helping critically ill patients very much. (*Not* I like very much helping critically ill patients)

We usually say the place before the time:

- She has been practicing interventional cardiology in *London* since *April*.

We put some adverbs in the middle of the sentence. If the verb is one word we put the adverb before the verb:

- I performed his stress test and *also spoke* to his family.

We put the adverb after *to be*:

- You *are always* on time.

We put the adverb after the first part of a compound verb:

- Are you *definitely attending* the stress-echo course?

In negative sentences we put probably before the negative:

- I *probably won't see* you at the congress.

We also use *all* and *both* in these positions:

- Jack and Tom are *both* able to carry out a coronary angiogram.
- We *all* felt sick after the meal.

Relative Clauses

A clause is a part of a sentence. A relative clause tells us which person or thing (or what kind of person or thing) the speaker means.

A relative clause (e.g., "Who is on call?") begins with a relative pronoun (e.g., *who, that, which, whose*).

A relative clause comes after a noun phrase (e.g., *the doctor, the nurse*).

Most relative clauses are defining clauses, and some of them are non-defining clauses.

Defining Clauses

- The book of interventional cardiology *(that) you lent to me is very interesting.*

The relative clause is essential to the meaning of the sentence.

Commas are not used to separate the relative clause from the rest of the sentence.

That is often used instead of *who* or *which*, especially in speech.

If the relative pronoun is the subject of the clause, it cannot be omitted.

Non-Defining Clauses

- The first ASD closure in Australia, *which took place at our hospital*, was a complete success.

The relative clause is not essential to the meaning of the sentence; it gives us additional information.

Commas are usually used to separate the relative clause from the rest of the sentence.

That cannot be used instead of *who* or *which*.

The relative pronoun cannot be omitted.

Relative Pronouns

Relative pronouns are used for people and for things.

- For people:
  - Subject: *who, that*
  - Object: *who, that, whom*
  - Possessive: *whose.*

- For things:
  - Subject: *which, that*
  - Object: *which, that*
  - Possessive: *whose.*

Who is used only for people. It can be the subject or the object of a relative clause:

- The patient *who was admitted in a shock situation* is getting better. Can we perform the echocardiogram now?

Which is used only for things. Like *who*, it can be the subject or object of a relative clause:

- The material, *which is used for resynchronization devices*, is very expensive.

That is often used instead of who or which, especially in speech.

Whom is used only for people. It is grammatically correct as the object of a relative clause, but it is very formal and is not often used in spoken English. We can use *whom* instead of *who* when *who* is the object of the relative clause, or when there is a preposition after the verb of the relative clause:

- The resident *who* I am going to the congress with is very nice.
  - The resident *with whom* I am going to the congress is a very nice and intelligent person.
- The patient *who* I saw in the Interventional Cardiology Service yesterday has been diagnosed with WPW syndrome.
  - The patient *whom* I saw in the Interventional Cardiology Service yesterday has been diagnosed with WPW syndrome.

Whose is the possessive relative pronoun. It can be used for people and things. We cannot omit *whose*:

- Nurses *whose* wages are low should be paid more.

We can leave out *who, which*, or *that*:

- When it is the object of a relative clause:
  - The article on the LBBB *that* you wrote is great.
  - The article on LBBB treatment you wrote is great.
- When there is a preposition. Remember that, in a relative clause, we usually put a preposition in the same place as in the main clause (after the verb):
  - The congress *that* we are going to next week is very expensive.
  - The congress we are going to next week is very expensive.

Prepositions in Relative Clauses

We can use a preposition in a relative clause with *who*, *which*, or *that*, or without a pronoun.

In relative clauses, we put a preposition in the same place as in a main clause (after the verb). We do not usually put it before the relative pronoun. This is the normal order in informal spoken English:

- This is a problem *which* we can do very little *about*.
- The nurse (*who*) I spoke *to* earlier isn't here now.

In more formal or written English, we can put a preposition at the beginning of a relative clause. But if we put a preposition at the beginning, we can only use *which* or *whom*. We cannot use the pronouns *that* or *who* after a preposition:

- This is a problem *about which* we can do very little.
- The nurse *to whom* I spoke earlier isn't here now.

Relative Clauses without a Pronoun (Special Cases)

Infinitive Introducing a Clause

We can use the infinitive instead of a relative pronoun and a verb after:

- The first, the second ... and the next
- The only
- Superlatives

For example:
- Roentgen was the *first* man to use X-rays.
- Joe was the *only* one to make the diagnosis.

-ing and -ed Forms Introducing a Clause

When we can use an *-ing* instead of a relative pronoun and an active verb:

- Residents *wanting to train abroad* should have a good level of English.

We can use an *-ed* form instead of a relative pronoun and a passive verb:

- The man *injured in the accident* was taken to the CT room.

The *-ing* form or the *-ed* form can replace a verb in a present or past tense.

Why, When, and Where

We can use *why*, *when*, and *where* in a defining relative clause.

We can leave out *why* or *when*. We can also leave out *where*, but then we must use a preposition.

We can form non-defining relative clauses with *when* and *where*:

- The clinical history, *where* everything about a patient is written, is a very important document.

We cannot leave out *when* and *where* from a non-defining clause.

Adjectives

An adjective describes (tells us something about) a noun.

In English, adjectives come before nouns (*old* hospital) and have the same form in both the singular and the plural (*new* hospital, *new* hospitals), and in the masculine and in the feminine.

An adjective can be used with certain verbs such as *be, get, seem, appear, look* (meaning seem), *feel, sound, taste* …:

- He has *been* ill since Friday, so he couldn't perform the angiogram.
- The patient *was* getting worse.
- The right ventricular biopsy *seemed* easy, but it wasn't.
- Free air in pneumothorax *appears* black on plain chest X-rays.

Adjective Order

We have fact adjectives and opinion adjectives. Fact adjectives (*large, new, white*) give us objective information about something (*size, age, color*). Opinion adjectives (*nice, beautiful, intelligent*) tell us what someone thinks of something.

In a sentence, opinion adjectives usually go before fact adjectives:

- An intelligent (*opinion*), young (*fact*) cardiologist visited me this morning.
- Dr. King has a nice (*opinion*), red (*fact*) Porsche.

Sometimes there are two or more fact adjectives describing a noun, and generally, we put them in the following order:

1. Size/length
2. Shape/width

3. Age
4. Color
5. Nationality
6. Material

For example:

- A *tall, young* nurse
- A *small, round* lesion
- A *black latex, leaded* pair of gloves
- A *large, new, white latex, leaded* pair of gloves
- An *old* American patient
- A *tall, young* Italian resident
- A *small, square, old, blue* iron monitor.

Regular Comparison of Adjectives

The form used for a comparison depends upon the number of syllables in the adjective.

Adjectives of One Syllable

One-syllable adjectives (for example, *fat, thin, tall*) are used with expressions of the form:

- Less … than (inferiority)
- As … as (equality)
- *-er* … than (superiority)

For example:

- The patient's condition was *less* severe *than* we had thought.
- Eating in the hospital is *as* cheap *as* eating at the medical school.
- Male patients' hearts tend to be big*ger than* female patients' ones.

Adjectives of Two Syllables

Two-syllable adjectives (for example, *easy, dirty, clever*) are used with expressions of the form:

- Less … than (inferiority)
- As … as (equality)
- *-er*/more … than (superiority).

We prefer *-er* for adjectives ending in *-y* (*easy, funny, pretty*) and other adjectives (such as *quiet, simple, narrow, clever*). For other two-syllable adjectives, we use *more*.

For example:

- The cardiovascular problem is *less* simple *than* you think.
- My chest is *as* painful *as* it was yesterday.
- The board exam was easi*er than* we expected.
- His illness was *more* serious *than* we first suspected.

Adjectives of Three or More Syllables

Adjectives of three or more syllables (for example *difficult, expensive, comfortable*) are used with expressions of the form:

- Less ... than (inferiority)
- As ... as (equality)
- More ... than (superiority)

For example:

- Studying medicine in Spain is *less* expensive *than* in the States.
- The small hospital was *as* comfortable *as* a hotel.
- Studying the case was *more* interesting *than* I had thought.

Before the comparative of adjectives, you can use:

- A (little) bit
- A little
- Much
- A lot
- Far

For example:

- I am going to try something *much* simpler to solve the problem.
- The patient is *a little* better today.
- The little boy is *a bit* worse today.

Sometimes it is possible to use two comparatives together (when we want to say something in changing continuously):

- It is becoming *more* and *more* difficult to find a job in an academic hospital.

We also say *twice as ... as, three times as ... as*:

- Going to the European Congress of Cardiology is *twice as* expensive *as* going to the French one.

The Superlative

The form used for a superlative depends upon the number of syllables in the adjective:

Adjectives of One Syllable

One-syllable adjectives are used with expressions of the form:

- The ...-*est*
- The least

For example:

- The number of cardiologist in your country is the high*est* in the world.

Adjectives of Two Syllables

Two-syllable adjectives are used with expressions of the form:

- The ...-*est*/the most
- The least

For example:

- The EKG is one of the *commonest* tests in clinical practice.
- The EKG is one of *the most* common tests in clinical practice.

Adjectives of Three or More Syllables

- The most
- The least

For example:

- Common sense and patience are *the most* important things for a cardiologist.
- This is *the least* difficult PTCA I have made in years.

Irregular Forms of Adjectives

- Good, better, the best
- Bad, worse, the worst
- Far, farther/further, the farthest/furthest

For example:

- My ultrasound technique is *worse* now than during my first year of residency, in spite of having attended several ultrasound refresher courses.

Comparatives with *The*

We use *the* + comparative to talk about a change in one thing that causes a change in something else:

- *The* nearer the X-ray focus, *the* better image we have.
- *The* more you practice ultrasound, *the* easier it gets.
- *The* higher the contrast amount, *the* greater the risk of renal failure.

As

Two things happening at the same time or over the same period of time:

- The resident listened carefully *as* Dr. Fraser explained to the patient the different diagnostic possibilities.
- I began to enjoy the residency more *as* I got used to being on call.

One thing happening during another:

- The patient died *as* the angioplasty was being performed.

Note that we use *as* only if two actions happen together. If one action follows another we don't use *as*, then we use the particle *when*:

- *When* the shocked patient came to the cath lab, I decided to call the surgeon.

Meaning *because*:

- *As* I was feeling sick, I decided to go to the doctor.

Like and *As*

Like

Like is a preposition, so it can be followed by a noun, pronoun or *-ing* form.

It means *similar to* or *the same as*. We use it when we compare things:

- What does he do? He is a cardiologist, *like* me.

As

As + subject + verb:

- Don't change the dose of contrast agent. Leave everything *as* it is.
- He should have been treated *as* I showed you.

As can have the meaning of *what*, as in the following example:

- The resident did *as* he was told.
- He made the diagnosis just with the chest X-ray, *as* I expected.
- *As* you know, we are sending an article to *Circulation* next week.
- *As* I thought, the patient was under the influence of alcohol.

As can also be a preposition, so it can be used with a noun, but it has a different meaning from *like*.

As + noun is used to say what something really is or was (especially when we talk about someone's job or how we use something):

- Before becoming a cardiologist I worked *as* a general practitioner in a small village.

As if, *as though* are used to say how someone or something looks, sounds, feels, etc., or to say how someone does something:

- The doctor treated me *as if* I were his son.
- John sounds *as though* he has got a cold.

Expressions with *as*:

- *Such as*
- *As usual* (Dr. Bombay was late *as usual*).

So and Such

So and *such* make the meaning of the adjective stronger.

We use *so* with an adjective without a noun or with an adverb:

- The first-year resident is *so clever*.
- The doctor injected lidocaine *so carefully* that the patient did not notice it.

We use *such* with an adjective with a noun:

- She is *such* a *clever resident*.

Prepositions

At/On/In Time

We use *at* with times:

- *At* 7 o'clock
- *At* midnight
- *At* breakfast time.

We usually leave out *at* when we ask (*at*) *what time*:

- *What time* are you working this evening?

We also use *at* in these expressions:

- *At* night
- *At* the moment
- *At* the same time
- *At* the beginning of
- *At* the end of

For example:

- I don't like to be on call *at night*.
- Dr. Artaiz is reporting some EKGs *at the moment*.

We use *in* for longer periods:

- *In* June
- *In* summer
- *In* 1977.

We also say *in the morning, in the afternoon, in the evening*:

- I'll finish all the pending discharge reports *in the morning*.

We use *on* with days and dates:

- *On* October 9th
- *On* Monday
- *On* Saturday mornings
- *On* the weekend (but "*at* the weekend" in British English).

We do not use *at/in/on* before *last* and *next*:

- I'll be on call *next* Saturday.
- They bought a new scanner *last* year.

We use *in* before a period (i.e., a time in the future):

• Our resident went to Boston to do a rotation on interventional cardiology. He'll be back *in* a year.

For, During, and While

We use *for* to say how long something takes:

• I've worked as a cardiologist at this hospital *for* 10 years.

You cannot use *during* in this way:

• It rained *for* 5 days (not *during* 5 days).

We use *during* + noun to say when something happens (not how long):

• The resident fell asleep *during* the stress-echo conference.

We use *while* + subject + verb:

• The resident fell asleep *while* he was attending the stress-echo conference.

By and Until

By + a time (i.e., not later than; you cannot use *until* with this meaning):

• I mailed the article on carotid dissection today, so they should receive it *by* Tuesday.

Until can be used to say how long a situation continues:

• Let's wait *until* the patient gets better.

When you are talking about the past, you can use *by the time*:

• *By the time* they got to the hotel the congress had already started.

In/At/On

We use *in* as in the following examples:

• *In* a room
• *In* a building
• *In* a town/*in* a country: "Dr. Concha works *in* Málaga."
• *In* the water/ocean/river.
• *In* a row
• *In* the hospital.

We use *at* as in the following examples:

- *At* the bus stop
- *At* the door/window
- *At* the top/bottom
- *At* the airport
- *At* work
- *At* sea
- *At* an event: "I saw Dr. Jules *at* the resident's party."

We use *on* as in the following examples:

- *On* the ceiling
- *On* the floor
- *On* the wall
- *On* a page
- *On* your nose
- *On* a farm.

In or At?

- We say *in the corner of a room*, but *at the corner of a street.*

- We say *in* or *at* college/school. Use *at* when you are thinking of the college/school as a place or when you give the name of the college/school:
  - Thomas will be *in* college for three more years.
  - He studied medicine *at* Harvard Medical School.

- With buildings, you can use *in* or *at.*

Arrive

We say:

- *Arrive in* a country or town: "Dr. Concha *arrived in* Boston yesterday."
- *Arrive at* other places: "Dr. Concha *arrived at* the airport a few minutes ago."

But, we omit in and at:

- *Arrived home.* "Dr. Concha *arrived* home late after sending the article to *Circulation.*"

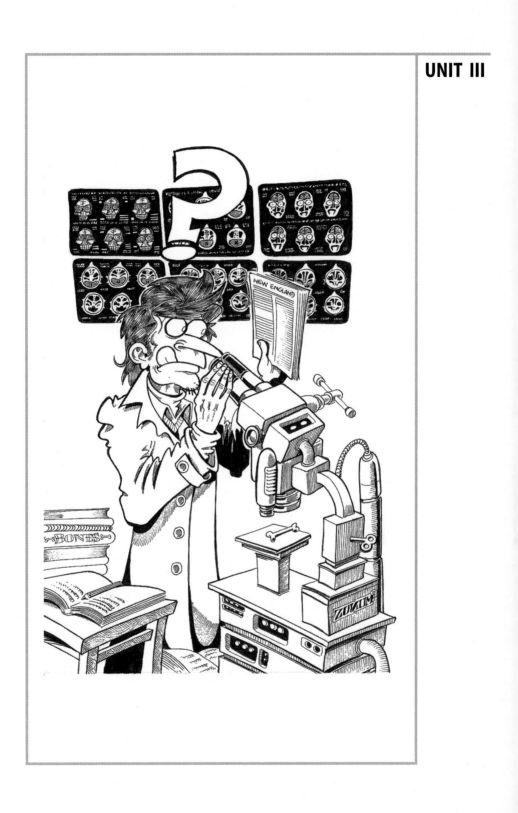

Unit III   Cardiovascular Scientific Literature: Writing an Article

Introduction

This chapter is not intended to be a "Guide for Authors," such as those that you can find in any journal. Our main advice is *not to write the paper first in your own language and then translate it into English; Instead, do it in English directly.*

Preliminary Work

When you have a subject that you want to report, first you need to look up references. You can refer to the *Index Medicus*® (http://www.ncbi.nlm.nih.gov/entrez/query.fcgi?db=PubMed) to search for articles. Once you have found them, read them thoroughly and underline those sentences or paragraphs that you think you might quote in your article.

Our advice is not to write the paper in your own language, but to do it directly in English. In order to do so, pick up, either out of these references, or out of the journal in which you want your work to be published, the article that you find closest to the type of study that you want to report.

Although you must follow the instructions of the journal to which you want to send the paper, here we use a standard form that may be adequate for most of them. In each section, we give you a few examples just to show how you can get them from other articles.

Article Header

Title

The title of the article should be concise but informative. Put a lot of thought into the title of your article.

Abstract

An abstract of 150–250 words (it depends on the journal) must be submitted with each manuscript. Remember that an abstract is a synopsis, not an introduction to the article.

The abstract should answer the question: "What should the reader know after reading this article?"

Most journals require that the abstract is divided into four paragraphs with the following headings.

Objective

State the purposes of the study or investigation; the hypothesis being tested or the procedure being evaluated.

Notice that very often you may construct the sentence beginning with an infinitive tense:

- *To evaluate* the impact of false positive lesions in coronary arteries studied with 64-multislice CT.
- *To present* our experience with septal embolization in hypertrophic cardiomyopathy.
- *To study* the diagnostic value of SPECT for left main coronary lesions.
- *To assess* stem cell intramyocardial injection after infarction.
- *To compare* the effect of flecainide vs amiodarone in patients with atrial fibrillation.
- *To determine* the prevalence of patency following angioplasty and to identify predictors of this patency.
- *To develop* an efficient and fully unsupervised method to quantitatively assess myocardial contraction from 4D-tagged MR sequences.
- *To investigate* the prognostic value of FDG PET uptake parameters in patients who undergo primary PTCA during AMI.
- *To ascertain* recent trends in imaging workload among the various medical specialties.
- *To describe* the clinical presentation and sonographic diagnosis of mitral valve prolapse.
- *To establish* ..., *To perform* ..., *To study* ..., *To design* ..., *To analyze* ..., *To test* ..., *To define* ..., *To illustrate* ..., etc.

You can also begin with "The aim/purpose/objective/goal of this study was to …":

> - *The aim of this study was to* determine the prognostic importance of viable myocardium in PET scan previous to CABG operation in patient with anterior myocardial infarction.
> - *The purpose of this study was* to compare feasibility and precision of renal artery stent placement using two different guidance techniques.
> - *The objective of this study was to* determine whether acute myocardial infarction (MI) can be diagnosed on contrast-enhanced helical chest CT.

You may give some background and then state what you have done:

> - *Viral pericarditis is an old clinical entity, which frequently mimics acute coronary syndromes, resulting in unnecessary admissions and tests. The purpose of this study was to describe CT-scan coronary findings in patients with acute pericarditis.*
> - *Myocardial fibrosis is known to occur in patients with hypertrophic cardiomyopathy (HCM) and to be associated with myocardial dysfunction. This study was designed to clarify the relation between myocardial fibrosis demonstrated by gadolinium-enhanced magnetic resonance imaging (Gd-MRI) and procollagen peptides or cytokines.*
> - *We hypothesized that …*
> - *We compared …*
> - *We investigated …*

Materials and Methods

Briefly state what was done and what materials were used, including the number of subjects. Also include the methods used to assess the data and to control bias.

> - N *patients with … were included.*
> - N *patients with … were excluded.*
> - N *patients known to have/suspected of having …*
> - *… was performed in N patients with …*
> - N *patients underwent …*
> - *Quantitative/qualitative analyses were performed by …*
> - *Patients were followed clinically for … months/years.*
> - *We examined the effects of iodinated IV contrast on blood pressure, heart rate, and renal function, after a CT scan in 15 healthy young volunteers.*

Results

Provide the findings of the study, including indicators of statistical significance. Include actual numbers, as well as percentages.

- *Twelve patients had acute myocardial infarction (AMI) and nine patients acute myocarditis (AM). All AMI but one displayed a territorial early subendocardial defect with corresponding delayed enhancement. All AMI displayed stenosis of at least the corresponding coronary artery. All AM but one displayed normal first-pass enhancement patterns and focal of diffuse non-territorial non-subendocardial delayed enhancement with normal coronary arteries in all cases.*
- *In our experience the mean reference vessel diameter by QCA was 3.81 ± 0.62 mm and a 3.5 mm or a 4 mm balloon were used in 33 and 35% of the cases respectively for pre-dilation. The mean final MLD was 3.93 ± 0.54 mm. A short (8–10 mm) LM was treated in 11% of cases, while a medium (10–15 mm) or a long (>15 mm) LM were treated in 25 and 64% of cases, respectively. The mean stented length in our series was of 15.5 ± 4.9 mm, and the ratio of lesion length to stented length was 0.64 ± 0.33.*
- *There was a tendency to a lower in-hospital mortality in patients treated with primary PTCA (2.6 vs 6.5%, p = 0.06). Non-fatal reinfarction or death during hospitalization was less frequent in patients treated with primary PTCA (5 vs 12%, p = 0.02). Intracranial bleeding was more frequent in patients treated with thrombolysis (2 vs 0%, p = 0.05). A re-do intervention necessity was higher in patients treated with thrombolysis, both by PTCA (36 vs 6%, p < 0.001) and by CABG (12 vs 8%, NS).*

Conclusion

Summarize in one or two sentences the conclusion(s) made on the basis of the findings. It should emphasize new and important aspects of the study or observations.

- *Diabetic patients remain a difficult cohort of patients to treat for the Interventional Cardiologist because of both increased periprocedural and follow-up adverse cardiac events.*
- *In-stent restenosis remains an ever increasing clinical problem for the interventional cardiologist, as the use of intracoronary stents continues to expand.*
- *With the intrinsic limitations of cardiac transplantation, cell transplantation is definitely a potential novel treatment strategy for patients with heart failure.*

- *Color-coded duplex ultrasonography has its fixed place in the evaluation of peripheral obstructive arterial disease. In calculating the degree of internal carotid stenosis it is as accurate as the gold standard of angiography.*
- *Cerebral protection will most likely decrease the complications rate of carotid stent procedures further, possibly turning this intervention into the therapy of choice for patients in whom carotid artery intervention is indicated.*
- *The study data demonstrate ..., Preliminary findings indicate ..., Results suggest ..., etc.*

Keywords

Below the abstract you should provide, and identify as such, three to ten keywords or short phrases that will assist indexers in cross-indexing the article and may be published with the abstract. The terms used should be from the "Medical Subject Headings" list of the *Index Medicus* (http://www.nlm.nih.gov/mesh/meshhome.html).

Main Text

The text of observational and experimental articles is usually (but not necessarily) divided into sections with the headings "Introduction," "Materials and Methods," "Results," and "Discussion." Long articles may need subheadings within some sections (especially the "Results and Discussion" sections) to clarify their content. Other types of articles such as case reports, reviews, and editorials, are likely to need other formats. You should consult individual journals for further guidance.

Avoid using abbreviations. When used, abbreviations should be spelled out the first time a term is given in the text, for example, "percutaneous transluminal coronary angioplasty (PTCA)."

Introduction

The text should begin with the "Introduction," which conveys the nature and purpose of the work and quotes the relevant literature. Give only strictly pertinent background information necessary for understanding why the topic is important and references that inform the reader as to why you undertook your study. Do not review the literature extensively. The final paragraph should clearly state the hypothesis or purpose of your study. Brevity and focus are important.

Materials and Methods

Details of clinical and technical procedures should follow the "Introduction." Describe your selection of the observational or experimental subjects (patients or laboratory animals, including controls) clearly. Identify the age, gender, and other important characteristics of the subjects. Because the relevance of such variables is not always clear, authors should explicitly justify them when they are included in a study report. The guiding principle should be clarity about how and why a study was done in a particular way. For example, authors should explain why only subjects of certain ages were included or why women were excluded. You should avoid terms such as "race," which lacks precise biological meaning, and use alternative concepts such as "ethnicity" or "ethnic group" instead. You should also specify carefully what the descriptors mean, and say exactly how the data were collected (for example, what terms were used in survey forms, whether the data were self-reported or assigned by others, etc.).

- *Our study population was selected from ...*
- *N patients underwent ...*
- *N consecutive patients ...*
- *N patients with proven ...*
- *Patients were followed clinically.*
- *N patients with ... were examined before and during ...*
- *N patients with known or suspected ... were prospectively enrolled in this study.*
- *More than N patients presenting with ... were examined with ... over a period of N months.*
- *N patients were prospectively enrolled between ... (date) and ... (date).*
- *N patients (N men, N women; age range N–N years; mean N.N years)*
- *In total, 140 patients, aged 50–70 years (mean 60 years), all with aortic valve sclerosis, were included in the study.*
- *Patients undergoing elective coronary angiogram for evaluation of chest pain were considered eligible if angiography documented ....*

Identify the methods, instrumentation (trade names and manufacturer's name and location in parentheses), and procedures in sufficient detail to allow other workers to reproduce your study. Identify precisely all drugs and chemical used, including generic name(s), dose(s), and route(s) of administration.

- *After baseline PET investigation, 40 mg of fluvastatin (Cranoc, Astra) was administered.*
- *MR imaging of the heart was performed with a 1.5-T system (Vision, Siemens, Erlangen, Germany).*
- *All patients underwent 16-row MSCT (Sensation 16, Siemens, Germany) with the following parameters: detector rows, 16; collimation, 0.75 mm; gantry rotation time, 375 ms.*
- *One hundred consecutive patients with atrial fibrillation and a ventricular rate above 135 bpm were randomized to receive either 450 mg of amiodarone or 0.6 mg of digoxin given as a single bolus through a peripheral venous access. If the ventricular rate exceeded 100 bpm after 30 min, then another 300 mg of amiodarone or 0.4 mg of digoxin were added. Primary endpoints of the study were the ventricular rate and the occurrence of sinus rhythm after 30 and 60 min. Secondary endpoints were blood pressure during the first hour after drug administration, and safety regarding drug induced hypotension, and phlebitis at the infusion site.*
- *We assessed epicardial patency according to the TIMI (thrombolysis in myocardial infarction) scale and myocardial patency according to the TMPG (TIMI myocardial perfusion grade) scale. In addition, we analyzed ST-segment resolution in 12-lead electrocardiography (EKG). The EKG was performed before and 30 min after PCI.*

It is essential that you state the manner by which studies were evaluated: independent readings, consensus readings, blinded or unblended to other information, time sequencing between readings of several studies of the same patient or animal to eliminate recall bias, random ordering of studies. It should be clear as to the retrospective or prospective nature of your study.

- *Entry/inclusion criteria included ...*
- *These criteria had to be met: ....*
- *Patients with ... were not included.*
- *Further investigations, including ... and ..., were also performed.*
- *We retrospectively studied N patients with ...*
- *The reviews were not blinded to the presence of ...*
- *The following patient inclusion criteria were used: age between 16 and 50 years and patent foramen ovale, absence of pulmonary hypertension, QP/QS more than 2 and signed informed consent with agreement to attend follow-up visits. The following exclusion criteria were used: significant tricuspid regurgitation, severe left atrium enlargement and poor right ventricular function.*

- *Two interventional cardiologists in consensus studied the following parameters on successive angiograms ...*
- *Both the interventional cardiologists and echocardiographers who performed the study and evaluated the results were blinded to drug administration.*
- *Histological samples were evaluated in a blinded manner by one of the authors and an outside expert in cardiac pathology.*

Give references to established methods, including statistical methods that have been published but are not well known; describe new or substantially modified methods, and give reasons for using these techniques and evaluate their limitations. Identify precisely all drugs and chemicals used, including generic name(s), dose(s), and route(s) of administration. Do not use drug's trade name unless it is directly relevant.

- *The imaging protocol included ...*
- *To assess objectively the severity of mitral stenosis, all patients were scored using the Wilkins criteria [23].*
- *The Amplatzer device used for ASD closure has been described elsewhere [12]; and consists of a ...*
- *Sprague-Dawley rats received 3-day oral pre-treatment with: (1) water; (2) low dose atorvastatin (ATV) (2 mg/kg/day); (3) cilostazol (CIL) (20 mg/kg/day); and (4) ATV+CIL. Rats underwent 30-min coronary artery occlusion and 4-h reperfusion, or hearts explanted for immunoblotting, without being subjected to ischemia. Area at risk (AR) was assessed by blue dye and IS by triphenyl tetrazolium chloride.*

Statistics

Describe statistical methods with enough detail to enable a knowledgeable reader with access to the original data to verify the reported results. Put a general description of methods in the "Materials and Methods" section. When data are summarized in the "Results" section, specify the statistical methods used to analyze them:

- *The statistical significance of differences was calculated with Fisher's exact test.*
- *The probability of ... was calculated using the Kaplan-Meier method.*
- *To test for statistical significance, ...*
- *Statistical analyses were performed with ... and ... tests.*
- *The levels of significance are indicated by p-values.*
- *Interobserver agreement was quantified by using K statistics.*

- *All p-values less than 0.05 were considered significant statistical indicators.*
- *Univariate and multivariate Cox proportional hazards regression models were used.*
- *The V^2 test was used for group comparison. Descriptive values of variables are expressed as means and percentages.*
- *We adjusted RRs for age (5-year categories) and used the Mantel extension test to test for linear trends. To adjust for other risk factors, we used multiple logistic regression.*

Give details about randomization:

- *They were selected consecutively by one physician between February 1999 and June 2000.*
- *This study was conducted prospectively during a period of 30 months from March 1998 to August 2000. WE enrolled 29 consecutive patients who had ...*

Specify any general-use computer programs used:

- *All statistical analyses were performed with SAS software (SAS Institute, Cary, N.C.).*
- *The statistical analyses were performed using a software package (SPSS for Windows, release 8.0; SPSS, Chicago, Ill).*

Results

Present your results in logical sequence in the text, along with tables, and illustrations. Do not repeat in the text all the data in the tables or illustrations; emphasize or summarize only important observations. Avoid nontechnical uses of technical terms in statistics such as "random" (which imply a randomizing device), "normal," "significant," "correlations," and "sample." Define statistical terms, abbreviations, and most symbols:

- *Statistically significant differences were shown for both X and X.*
- *Significant correlation was found between X and X.*
- *Results are expressed as means ± SD.*
- *All the abnormalities in our patient population were identified on the prospective clinical interpretation.*
- *The abnormalities were correctly characterized in 12 patients and incorrectly in ...*

- *The preoperative and operative characteristics of these patients are listed in Table X.*
- *The results of the US-guided ASD-closure are shown in Table X.*
- *The clinical findings are summarized in Table X.*

Report any complication:

- *Two minor complications were encountered. After the second procedure, one patient had a slight hemoptysis that did not require treatment, and one patient had chest pain for about 2 h after the stenting procedure.*
- *Among the 11 000 patients, there were 373 in-hospital deaths (3.4%), 204 intraoperative/postoperative CVAs (1.8%), 353 patients with postoperative bleeding events (3.2%), and 142 patients with sternal wound infections (1.3%).*

Give numbers of observations. Report losses to observation (such as dropouts from a clinical trial):

- *The final study cohort consisted of ...*
- *Of the 961 patients included in this study, 69 were reported to have died (including 3 deaths identified through the NDI), and 789 patients were interviewed. For 81 surviving patients, information was obtained from another source. Twenty-two patients (2.3%) could not be contacted and were not included in the analyses because information on nonfatal events was not available.*

Discussion

Within this section, use ample subheadings. Emphasize the new and important aspects of the study and the conclusions that follow from them. Do not repeat in detail data or other material given in the "Introduction" or "Results" sections. Include in the "Discussion" section the implications of the findings and their limitations, including implications for future research. Relate the observations to other relevant studies.

Link the conclusions with the goals of the study, but avoid unqualified statements and conclusions not completely supported by the data. In particular, avoid making statements on economic benefits and costs unless the report includes economic data and analyses. Avoid claiming priority and alluding to work that has not been completed. State new hypotheses when warranted, but clearly label them as such. Recommendations, when appropriate, may be included.

- *In conclusion, ...*
- *In summary, ...*
- *This study demonstrates that ...*
- *This study found that ...*
- *This study highlights ...*
- *Another finding of our study is ...*
- *One limitation of our study was ...*
- *Other methodological limitations of this study ...*
- *Our results support ...*
- *Further research is needed to elucidate ...*
- *However, the limited case number warrants a more comprehensive study to confirm these findings and to assess the comparative predictive value of ...*
- *Some follow-up is probably appropriate for these patients.*
- *Further research is needed when ... is available.*

Acknowledgments

List all contributors who do not meet the criteria for authorship, such as a person who provided purely technical help, writing assistance, or a department chair who provided only general support. Financial and material support should also be acknowledged.

People who have contributed materially to the paper but whose contributions do not justify authorship may be listed under a heading such as "clinical investigators" or "participating investigators," and their function or contribution should be described, for example, "served as scientific advisors," "critically reviewed the study proposal," "collected data," or "provided and cared for study patients,"

Because readers may infer their endorsement of the data and conclusions, everybody must have given written permission to be acknowledged.

- *The authors express their gratitude to ... for their excellent technical support.*
- *The authors tank Wei J. Chen, M.D., Sc.D., Institute of Epidemiology, College of Public Health, National Taiwan University, Taipei, for the analysis of the statistics and his help in the evaluation of the data. The authors also thank Pan C. Yang, D, Ph.D., Department of Internal Medicine, and Keh S. Tsai, M.D., Ph.D., Department of Laboratory Medicine, National Taiwan University, Medical College and Hospital, Taipei, for the inspiration and discussion of the research idea of this study. We also thank Ling C. Shen for her assistance in preparing the manuscript.*

References

References should be numbered consecutively in the order in which they are first mentioned in the text. Identify references in text, tables and legends by Arabic numerals in parentheses (some journals require superscript Arabic numbers). References cited only in tables or figure legends should be numbered in accordance with the sequence established by the first citation in the text of the particular table or figure.

- *Clinically, resting thallium-201 single-photon emission computed tomography (SPECT) has been widely used to evaluate myocardial viability in patients with chronic coronary arterial disease and acute myocardial infarction [8–16].*
- *In addition, we have documented a number of other parameters previously shown to exhibit diurnal variation, including an assessment of sympathetic activity, as well as inflammatory markers recently shown to relate to endothelial function.[14]*

Use the style of the examples below, which are based on the formats used by the National Library of Medicine (NLM) in *Index Medicus*. The titles of journals should be abbreviated according to the style used in *Index Medicus*. Consult the *List of Journals Indexed in Index Medicus*, published annually as a separate publication by the library and as a list in the January issue of *Index Medicus*. The list can also be obtained through the library's website (http://www.nlm.nih.gov).

Avoid using abstracts as references. References to papers accepted but not yet published should be designated as "in press" or "forthcoming"; authors should obtain written permission to cite such papers as well as verification that they have been accepted for publication. Information from articles submitted but not accepted should be cited in the text as "unpublished observations" with written permission from the source.

Avoid citing a "personal communication" unless it provides essential information not available from a public source, in which case the name of the person and date of communication should be cited in parentheses in the text. For scientific articles, authors should obtain written permission and confirmation of accuracy from the source of a personal communication.

The references must be verified by the author(s) against the original documents.

The Uniform Requirements style (the Vancouver style; http://www.icmje.org/) is based largely on an ANSI standard style adapted by the NLM for its databases (http://www.nlm.nih.gov/bsd/uniform_requirements.html). Notes have been added where Vancouver style differs from the style now used by NLM.

Articles in Journals

Standard Journal Article

List the first six authors followed by et al. (note: NLM now lists up through 25 authors; if there are more than 25 authors, NLM lists the first 24, then the last author, then et al.)

> *Van Belle E, Abolmaali K, Bauters C, McFadden EP, Lablanche JM, Bertrand ME. Restenosis, late vessel occlusion and left ventricular function six months after balloon angioplasty in diabetic patients. J Am Coll Cardiol 1999 Jun; 34(6):476–485*

As an option, if a journal carries continuous pagination throughout a volume (as many medical journals do) the month and issue number may be omitted. (Note: for consistency, the option is used throughout the examples in Uniform Requirements. NLM does not use the option.)

> *Van Belle E, Abolmaali K, Bauters C, McFadden EP, Lablanche JM, Bertrand ME. Restenosis, late vessel occlusion and left ventricular function six months after balloon angioplasty in diabetic patients. J Am Coll Cardiol 1999; 34:476–485*

Organization as Author

> *American Diabetes Association. Standards for medical care for patients with diabetes mellitus. Diabetes Care 2002; 25:S33–S49*

No Author Given

> *Cancer in South Africa (editorial). S Afr Med J 1994; 84:15*

Article Not in English

(Note: NLM translates the title to English, encloses the translation in square brackets, and adds an abbreviated language designator.)

> *Vogl TJ, Diebold T, Hammerstingl R, Balzer JO, Hidajat N, Zipfel B, Scheinert D, Vogt A, Beier J, Felix R. [Diagnostic of the abdominal vascular system with electronic beam CT (EBT)]. Radiologe 1998; 38:1069–176. German*

Volume with Supplement

> *Feener EP, King GL. Vascular dysfunction in diabetes mellitus. Lancet 1997; 350(Suppl1):9–13*

Issue with Supplement

> *Morris JJ, Smith LR, Jones RH, et al. Influence of diabetes and mammary artery grafting on survival after coronary bypass. Circulation 1991; 84 Suppl 3:III-275–284.*

Volume with Part

> *Ozben T, Nacitarhan S, Tuncer N. Plasma and urine sialic acid in non-insulin dependent diabetes mellitus. Ann Clin Biochem 1995; 32 (pt 3): 303–306*

Issue with Part

> *Poole GH, Mills SM. One hundred consecutive cases of flap lacerations of the leg in ageing patients. N Z Med J 1994; 107 (986 pt 1):377–378*

Issue with No Volume

> *Turan I, Wredmark T, Fellander-Tsai L. Arthroscopic ankle arthrodesis in rheumathoid arthritis. Clin Orthop 1995; (320):110–114*

No Issue or Volume

> *Browell DA, Lennard TW. Immunologic status of the cancer patient and the effects of blood transfusion on antitumor responses. Curr Opin Gen Surg 1993; 325–333*

Pages in Roman Numerals

> *Fisher GA, Sikic BI. Drug resistance in clinical oncology and haematology. Introduction. Hematol Oncol Clin North Am 1995 Apr; 9(2):xi–xii*

Type of Article Indicated as Needed

Alonso JJ, Fernandez-Aviles MF, Duran JM et al. Influence of diabetes mellitus on the initial and long-term outcome of patients treated with coronary stenting. J Am Coll Cardiol 1998; 31:(Suppl A)415A(abstr)
Ezensberger W, Fischer PA. Metronome in Parkinson's disease (letter). Lancet 1996; 347:1337

Article Containing Retraction

Garey CE, Schwarzman AL, Rise ML, Seyfried TN. Ceruloplasmin gene defect associated with epilepsy in EL mice [retraction of Garey CE, Schwarzman AL, Rise ML, Seyfried TN. In: Nat Genet 1994; 6:426–431]. Nat Genet 1995; 11:104

Article Retracted

Liou GI, Wang M, Matragoon S. Precocious IRBP gene expression during mouse development [retracted in Invest Ophthalmol Vis Sci 1994; 35:3127]. Invest Ophtalmol Vis Sci 1994; 35:108–138

Article with Published Erratum

Hamlin JA, Kahn AM. Herniography in symptomatic patients following inguinal hernia repair [published erratum appears in West J Med 1995; 162:278]. West J Med 1995; 162:28–31

Books and Other Monographs

Personal Author(s)

Waller BF. Cardiac Morphology. 1st ed. Philadelphia: Saunders Company, 1984

Editors(s), Compiler(s) as Author

Giuliani ER, Gersh BJ, McGoon M.D., Hayes DL, Schaff HV. Mayo clinic practice of cardiology. 3rd ed. St. Louis. Mosby-Year Book, Inc. 1996

Conference Proceedings

Scheinert D, Rag JC, Vogt A, Biamino G. In: Henry M, Amor M. (eds) Excimer Laser Assisted Recanalization of Chronic Arterial Occlusions. Ninth International Course Book of Peripheral Vascular Interventions 1998; 139–155

Kimura J, Shibasaki H, editors. Recent advances in clinical neurophysiology. Proceedings of the 10th International Congress of EMG and Clinical Neurophysiology; 1995 Oct 15–19; Kyoto, Japan. Amsterdam: Elsevier; 1996

Organization as Author and Publisher

Institute of Medicine (US). Looking at the future of the Medicaid program. Washington: The Institute; 1992

Chapter in a Book

Redfield MM. Evaluation of congestive heart failure. In: Guiliani ER, Gersh BJ, McGoon M.D., Hayes DL, Schaff HV editors. Mayo clinic practice of cardiology. 3rd ed. St. Louis. Mosby-Year Book, Inc. 1996

Conference Paper

Bengtsson S, Solheim BG. Enforcement of data protection, privacy and security in medical informatics. In: Lun KC, Deoulet P, Piemme TE, Rienhoff O, editors. MEDINFO 92. Proceedings of the 7th World Congress on Medical Informatics; 1992 Sep 6–10; Geneva, Switzerland. Amsterdam: North-Holland; 1992. pp. 1561–1565

Scientific or Technical Report

Issued by Funding/Sponsoring Agency

Smith P, Golladay K. Payment for durable medical equipment billed during skilled nursing facility stays. Final report. Dallas (TX): Dept. of Health and Human Services (US) office of Evaluation and Inspections; 1994 Oct. Report No. HHSIGOEI69200860

Issued by Performing Agency

Field MJ, Tranquada RE; Feasley JC, editors. Health services research: work force and educational issues. Washington: National Academy Press; 1995. Contract No. AHCPR282942008. Sponsored by the Agency for Health Care Policy and Research

Dissertation

Kaplan SJ. Post-hospital home health care: the elderly's access and utilization [dissertation]. St. Louis (MO): Washington Univ.; 1995

Patent

Larsen CE, Trip R, Johnson CR, inventors; Novoste Corporation, assignee. Methods for procedures related to the electrophysiology of the heart. US patent 5,529,067. 1995 Jun 25

Other Published Material

Newspaper Article

Lee G. Hospitalization tied to ozone pollution: study estimates 50,000 admissions annually. The Washington Post 1996 Jun 21; Sect. A:3(col. 5)

Audiovisual Material

HIV+/AIDS: the facts and the future [videocassette]. St. Louis (MO): Mosby-Year Book; 1995

Dictionary and Similar References

Stedman's medical dictionary. 26th ed. Baltimore: Williams&Wilkins;1995. Apraxia; pp. 119–120

Unpublished Material

In Press

(Note: NLM prefers "forthcoming" because not all items will be printed.)

Maehara A, Mintz GS, Castagna MT, et al. Intravascular ultrasound assessment of spontaneous coronary artery dissection. Am J Cardiol (in press).
Assessment of chest pain in the emergency room: What is the role of multidetector CT? Eur J Radiol. In press 2006

Electronic Material

Journal Article in Electronic Format

Morse SS. Factors in the emergence of infectious diseases. EMerg Infect Dis [serial online] 1995 Jan–Mar [cited 1996 Jun 5];1(1):[24 screens]. Available from: URL:http://www.cdc.gov/ncidod/EID/eid.htm

Monograph in Electronic Format

CDI, clinical dermatology illustrated [monograph on CD-ROM]. Reeves JRT, Maibach H. CMEA Multimedia Froup, producers. 2nd ed. Version 2.0. San Diego: CMEA; 1995

Computer File

Hemodynamics III: the ups and downs of hemodynamics [computer program]. Version 2.2. Orlando (FL): Computerized Educational Systems; 1993

Additional Material

Tables

All tabulated data identified as tables should be given a table number and a descriptive caption. Take care that each tale is cited in numerical sequence in the text.

The presentation of data and information given in the table headings should not duplicate information already given in the text. Explain in footnotes all non-standard abbreviations used in the table.

If you need to use any table or figure from another journal, make sure you ask for permission and put a note such as:

Adapted, with permission, from reference 5.

Figures

Figures should be numbered consecutively in the order in which they are first cited in the text. Follow the patterns of similar illustrations of your references.

- *Figure 1. Non-enhanced CT scan shows ...*

- *Figure 2. Contrast-enhanced CT scan obtained at the level of ...*

- *Figure 3. Selective coronary angiogram shows ...*

- *Figure 4. Photograph of a fresh-cut specimen shows ...*

- *Figure 5. Photomicrograph (original magnification, ×10; hematoxylin-eosin stain) of ...*

- *Figure 6. Parasternal short axis view of ...*

- *Figure 7. Typical flow-pattern in a 65-year-old female. (a) Four-chamber apical view shows ...*

- *Figure 8. Shows the results after the stent implantation. A large proximal dissection was noted and a 3 by 32 mm in length NIR primo stent was placed proximally, deployed at 10 ATM.*

- *Figure 9. Ostial left main stenosis before and after stenting. LAD contains a mid segment aneurysm which was covered with a Jomed covered stent graft.*

Final Tips

Before you submit your article for publication check its spelling, and go over your article for words you might have omitted or typed twice, as well as words you may have misused such as using "there" instead of "their." Do not send an article with spelling or dosage errors or other medical inaccuracies. And do not expect the spell-check function on your computer to catch all your spelling mistakes.

Be accurate. Check and double-check your facts and reference citations. Even after you feel the article is finished leave it for a day or two and then go back to it. The changes you make to your article after seeing it in a new light will often be the difference between a good article and a great article.

Once you believe everything is correct, give the draft to your English teacher for a final informal editing. Do not send your first (or even second) draft to the publisher!

Do not forget to read and follow carefully the specific "Instructions for Authors" of the journal in which you want your work to be published.

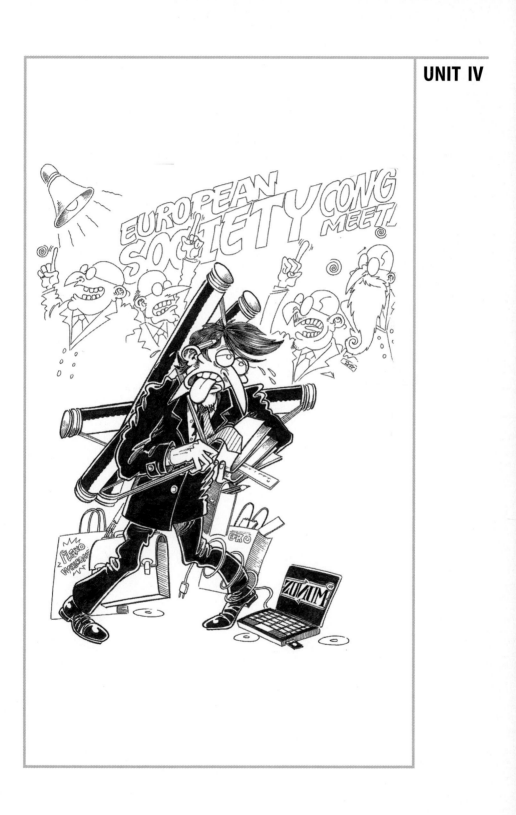

Unit IV Letters to Editors of Cardiovascular Journals

Introduction

This unit is made up of several examples of letters sent to editors of cardiovascular journals. Our intention is to provide you with useful tools to communicate with journal editors and reviewers in a formal manner. It is our understanding that letters to editors have quite an important, and many times overlooked, role in the fate of scientific cardiological manuscripts.

Although we are not going to focus on letters from editors since they are, generally speaking, easy to understand, these letters can be divided into acceptance "under certain conditions" letters, acceptance letters, and rejection letters:

- Acceptance "under certain conditions" letters. These letters, are relatively common, and usually mean a great deal of work since the paper must be re-written.
- Acceptance letters. Congratulations! Your paper has finally been accepted and no corrections have to be made. These letters are, unfortunately, relatively uncommon, and quite easy to read. Besides, they do not need to be replied to.
- Rejection letters. There are many polite formulas of letting you know that your paper is not going to be published in a particular journal. These letters are instantly understood and since they do not need to be replied to, no time needs to be wasted on them from an idiomatic point of view.

We have divided up the letters to editors into:

1. Submission letters
2. Resubmission letters
3. Reconfiguration letters
4. Letters of thanks for an invitation to publish an article in a journal
5. Letters asking about the status of a paper
6. Other letters

Submission Letters

Submission letters are quite easy to write since the only message to be conveyed is the type of the paper you are submitting and the name of the corresponding author. Many standard letters can be used for this purpose, and we do not think you have to waste too much time on them since they are mere preliminary material that just needs to be sent along with the paper itself.

Your address   Date

Receiver's name and address

Dear Dr. Alfonso,

Please find enclosed (*N*) copies of our manuscript entitled ".." (authors ..., ..., ...), which we hereby submit for publication in the ... Journal of ... Also enclosed is a diskette with a copy of the text file in Microsoft Word for Windows (version ...).

I look forward to hearing from you.

Yours sincerely,

A. J. Stephenson, M.D.

Resubmission Letters

Resubmission letters must thoroughly address the comments and suggestions of acceptance letters. It is in these letters where the corresponding author must let the editor know that all or at least most of the suggested changes have been made and, in doing so, the paper could be ready for publication. These letters may play quite an important role in the acceptance or rejection of a paper. Sometimes a lack of fluency in English prevents the corresponding author conveying the corrections made in the manuscript and the reasons why other suggested changes were not made.

Let us review the following example:

Dear Dr. Ho,

After a thorough revision in light of the reviewers' comments, we have decided to submit our paper "Radiofrequency Ablation for Atypical Atrial Flutter in The Elderly" for re-evaluation.

First of all, we would like to thank you for this second chance to present our paper for publication in your journal.

The main changes in the paper are related to your major comments:
– To describe precisely the endocardial mapping.
– To indicate what the clinical status of patients was.
– To include long-term follow up data and electric outcome.

Following your advice, we have also included changes that are in accordance with the reviewers' comments.

We hope this new revision will now be suitable for publication in your journal.

Yours sincerely,

Ignacio García Bolao, M.D., and co-authors

Reconfiguration Letters

Sometimes the paper is accepted provided its configuration is changed, i.e., from a pictorial review to a pictorial essay. Reconfiguration letters are resubmission letters as well and, therefore, tend to be long.

Review this example from which we have extracted and highlighted several sentences that can help you in your correspondence with journals.

"Predictors of early morbidity and mortality after thrombolytic therapy of acute myocardial infarction" RE:01–1243

Dear Dr. Moliterno, (1)

We have reconfigured the manuscript referenced above (2) in the form of a Pictorial Essay *following your suggestion (3)* and we have made as many changes as possible with regard to the reviewers' recommendations taking into account the *space limitation imposed by the new format of the paper (4)*.

We have tried to cover all aspects involving myocardial infarction, focusing on their more characteristic prognostic features and *giving priority to the most frequent complications of thrombolysis (5)*. The reconfiguration of the manuscript has shortened it so drastically that we have had to rewrite it entirely and *for this reason we do not attach an annotated copy (6) – if you still consider this necessary we will include it (7)*. Although tables are not permitted in pictorial essays, we think that the inclusion of a single table on the classification of available thrombolytics would *"allow the reader to more easily categorize the described complications (8)* as stated by reviewer no. 2 (9)* in his general remarks. The table has not been included due to the new format of the paper, but *if you take our suggestion into consideration we will be pleased to add it (10)*.

The major changes in our manuscript are:

1. *The title has been modified to* "Analysis of Outcome after Thrombolytic Therapy in AMI," *following your recommendation (11)*.
2. *We have included the EKG's findings*, although it has not been possible to expand the angiographic findings *as suggested by reviewer no. 1 (12)* due to space limitation.
3. *Similarly*, the description of thrombus containing lesions and TIMI flow *could not be expanded as suggested by reviewer no. 2 due to space limitation (13)*.
4. *With regard to figures (14):*
   a. We have included three new figures.
   b. *Precordial and limb leads on a given EKG have been included (15)*, as suggested, in figures 4, 7, 11, and 12.
   c. *The image quality of figure 3 has been improved (16)*.

5. We have assigned distinct figures to different entities in most cases although the limited number of figures allowed – 15 – made it impossible to do it in all cases.

6. *With regard to comments on figures by reviewer no. 1 (17):*

   a. Figure 4e is indeed an endocardial contrast enhanced echo (18). Inferior segment is not well seen due to the poor window in this obese patient, which was one of our first patients and needed to be included in the study.

   b. *Figure 5b shows an artifact due to an aortic prosthesis that had been implanted in the patient years ago (19).*

We look forward to hearing from you, (20)

Yours sincerely, (21)

Peter Berglar, M.D., and co-authors (22)

1. *Dear Dr. Moliterno,*
   – This sentence ends with a comma rather than a semicolon.

2. *We have reconfigured the manuscript referenced above …*
   – The content of the letter must be summarized in the first paragraph.

3. *… following your suggestion …*
   – This is one of the most common sentences in resubmission/reconfiguration letters.

4. *… space limitation imposed by the new format of the paper …*
   – Space limitation, provided the new format limits it, and must be taken into consideration by both the authors and the reviewers.

5. *… giving priority to the most prevalent conditions …*
   – May be a criterion for the shortening of the manuscript.

6. *… for this reason we do not attach an annotated copy …*
   – Whenever you do not follow a suggestion, you must give an explanation.

7. *… if you still consider it necessary we will include it …*
   – Always leave open the possibility of adding more information in further correspondence.

8. *… allow the reader to more easily categorize the described complications …*
   – You can use as an argument what was literally suggested by the reviewer by writing it in inverted commas.

9. *… as stated by reviewer no. 2 …*
   – This is a usual way of addressing a reviewer's comment.

10. *... if you take our suggestion into consideration we will be pleased to add it. ...*
    - This sentence can be used whenever you want to include something that has not been requested by the reviewers.
11. *The title has been modified to ... following your recommendation.*
    - This is a usual way of addressing a reviewer's comment.
12. *We have included our EKG's findings as suggested by reviewer no. 1 ...*
    - This is a usual way of addressing a reviewer's comment.
13. *Similarly, ... could not be expanded as suggested by reviewer no. 2 due to space limitations.*
    - Whenever you do not follow a suggestion, you must give an explanation.
14. *With regard to figures:*
    - Or *regarding figures, as regards figures, as for figures* (without the preposition "to")
15. *Precordial and limb leads on a given EKG have been included ...*
    - This is a usual way of addressing a reviewer's comment.
16. *The image quality of figure 3 has been improved ...*
    - This is a usual way of addressing a reviewer's comment.
17. *With regard to comments on figures by reviewer no. 1...*
18. *Figure 4e is indeed an endocardial-contrast enhanced echo*
19. *Figure 5b shows an artifact due to an aortic prosthesis that had been implanted in the patient years ago*
    - This is a usual way of addressing a reviewer's comment.
20. *We look forward to hearing from you,*
    - Remember that the verb following the verb phrase *to look forward to* must be in its *-ing* form.
21. *Peter Berglar, M.D., and co-authors*
    - Although the corresponding author is the only one who signs the letter, sometimes a reference is made to the co-authors.

Letters of Thanks for an Invitation to Publish an Article in a Journal

These are simple and usually short letters in which we let the editor of a journal know how pleased we are regarding his/her invitation and how much we appreciate his/her consideration.

Your address   Date

Receiver's name and address

Dear Dr. Scott,

Thank you for the invitation to submit a manuscript on coronary vulnerable plaques to your journal.

Please find attached our paper which details our imaging, diagnosis, and treatment protocols, and makes a thorough revision on the literature on the subject.

I look forward to hearing from you.

Yours sincerely,

S. V. Johnson, M.D.

Asking about the Status of a Paper

In these letters we inquire about the situation of our article, since we have not received any response from the journal. Regrettably in the academic world "no news" is not usually "good news," and many of these inquiries end up with a polite rejection letter.

Dear Dr. Fuster,

As I have not received any response regarding the manuscript "Baseline EKG Changes in Professional Cyclists," I am interested in obtaining some information on the status of the paper.

Please, use the following e-mail address for further correspondence: samedi@daytime.net

I look forward to hearing from you at your earliest convenience,

S. Medina, M.D., Ph.D.

Other Letters

Applying for a Post

11 St Albans Road
London SW17 5TZ

17 November 2006

Medical Staffing Officer
Brigham and Women's Hospital
18 Francis St.
Boston, MA 02115, USA

Dear Sir/Madam,

I wish to apply for the post of Consultant Non-invasive Cardiologist as advertised in the *Journal of the American College of Cardiology* of 22 November.

I enclose my CV and the names of two referees as requested.

Yours faithfully,

Felipe Mesa, M.D.

Asking for Permission to Use Someone's Name as a Referee

Platero Heredia, 19
Córdoba 14012
SPAIN

17 April 2006

Mark C. Fishman, M.D.
Department of Cardiology
Massachusetts General Hospital
22 Beacon St
Boston, MA 02114, USA

Dear Dr. Fishman,

I am applying for a post of Consultant Cardiologist at Cleveland Clinic. I should be most grateful if you allow me to use your name as a referee.

Yours sincerely,

Juan Pastrana, M.D.

Postponing the Commencement of Duties

Gran Vía, 113
Madrid, 28004
Spain

17 November 2006

Stephen N. Oesterle, M.D.
Department of Cardiology
Massachusetts General Hospital
22 Beacon St
Boston, MA 02114, USA

Dear Dr. Oesterle,

I would like to thank you for your letter of 11 February 2001, offering me the post of Consultant Cardiologist from 12 March 2005.

I am very pleased to accept the post but unfortunately I will not be able to arrive in Boston until 25 March 2005 due to personal reasons. Would it, therefore, be possible for you to postpone the commencement of my duties to 26 March 2005?

I look forward to hearing from you.

Yours sincerely,

María Spiteri, M.D.

In Summary

To sum up, a few simple formal details must be recalled:

- "Dear Dr. Smith," is the usual way to begin an academic letter. Recall that after the name of the editor, you must insert a comma instead of a semicolon, and continue the letter with a new paragraph.
- The usual formula "find enclosed ..." can nowadays be replaced by "find attached ...," talking into consideration that most papers are submitted via the internet.
- "I look forward to hearing from you," is a standard sentence at the end of any formal letter, and you have to bear in mind, in order to avoid a usual mistake, that "to" is a preposition to be followed by a gerund rather than the infinitive particle of the verb that follows it. Do not make the usual mistake of writing "I look forward to hear from you." Similar formulas are: "I look forward to receiving your comments on ...," "Very truly yours,"
- "Your consideration is appreciated" or "Thanks you for your and the reviewers' consideration" are standard sentences to be written at the end of letters to editors.
- "I look forward to receiving your feedback on ..." is a bit more casual formula commonly used in letters to editors.
- "Yours faithfully," is used when you do not know the name of the person you are writing to, whereas "Sincerely," "Sincerely yours," "Yours sincerely," or "Very truly yours," must be written when you address the letter to a person by name. Therefore, if the letter begins with "Dear Dr. Olsen," it must end up with "Yours sincerely," and if it is addressed to the editor as such it must finish with "Yours faithfully,." Don't forget that after the adverb or the pronoun, you must insert a comma, rather than a period, and, then, your signature below.
- Whenever you cannot address one of the editors' suggestions, explain why it was not possible in the resubmission letter so the reviewers do not waste time looking for it in the manuscript.

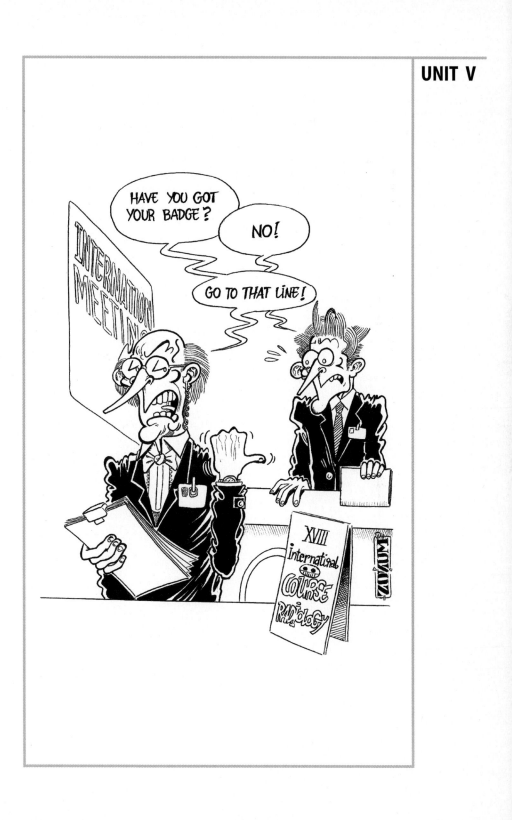

Unit V   Attending an International Cardiovascular Course

Introduction

In the following pages, we take a look inside international cardiological meetings. We recommend upper-intermediate English speakers to go over them quickly, and intermediate English speakers to review this section thoroughly in order to become familiar with the jargon of international congresses and that of the conversational scenarios such as the airport, plane, customs, taxi, hotel checking-in, and finally, the course itself that make up the usual itinerary of a cardiologist attending an international course.

Most beginners do not go alone to their first courses abroad. This fact, which in principle is a relief since they do not have to cope with the idiomatic difficulties on their own, has an important drawback: Most non–native English-speaking cardiology residents come back to their respective countries, without having uttered a single word in English. Although it may be considered quite unnatural, to speak in English with your colleagues is the only way of speaking in English during the course, since over 90% of your conversations are going to be those you have with your fellow countrymen. In parties of more than two people, it is virtually impossible to do this simple exercise.

Traveling alone is the only way of speaking English during an international cardiological course and, for a non–native English-speaking cardiologist, may be the only opportunity of keeping their English alive throughout the year. Do not waste this excellent opportunity to maintain your level of both colloquial English and cardiological English.

The following anecdote illustrates the level of uncertainty young non–native English-speaking doctors face when they attend their first international meetings. It was my first European Congress in Vienna. When I was expecting to be attended to at the registration desk and given my congress bag, somebody asked me, "Have you got your badge?" Not knowing what badge meant I said "no," since I was unlikely to have something on me I did not even know the name of. The next sentence I heard was uttered in a very commanding voice, "Go to that line!" so I obediently got into the line without knowing what on earth I was going to get from it. This was the first, but not the last, time I was in a line without having the slightest idea of what I was going to get from it. When this happens to you and you are supposed to give a lecture on, let's say, cardiomyopathies your desire to come back home is all that remains intact in you.

Do not let your lack of fluency in day-to-day English undermine your ability to deliver a good presentation. Colloquial English and cardiological English are two different worlds, and in order to be successful in the latter you must have a sound knowledge in the former.

This chapter provides you with tips and useful sentences in your itinerary to an international cardiology course: airport, plane, customs, taxi, hotel checking in, and finally, the course itself. Unless you have overcome the conversational hurdles in the scenarios that come before the course, first, you are not going to get to the course venue and, second, if you do get to it you will not feel like delivering your presentation.

Most non–native English-speaking lecturers resign themselves to just giving the lecture and "survive," forgetting that if they do not enjoy their lecture, the audience will not enjoy it either. They think that to enjoy giving a lecture, your native tongue must be English. We strongly disagree with this point since many speakers do not enjoy their talks in their own native tongues, and it is our understanding that having a good time delivering a presentation has much more to do with your personality than with your native tongue.

Travel and Hotel Arrangements

Airport

Getting to the Airport

- How can I get to the airport?
- How soon should we be at the airport before take-off?

Checking in

- *May I have your passport and flight tickets, please?* Of course, here you are.
- *Are you Mr. Macaya?* Right, I am. *How do you spell it?* M-A-C-A-Y-A. (Rehearse the spelling of your last name since if it is not an English one, you are going to be asked about its spelling many times).
- *Here is your boarding pass. Your flight leaves from gate 14.* Thank you.
- *You are only allowed two carry-on items. You'll have to check in that larger bag.*

Questions a Passenger Might Ask

- I want to fly to London leaving this afternoon. Is there a direct flight? Is it via Amsterdam?
- Is it direct? *Yes, it is direct./No, it has one stop.*
- Is there a layover? *Yes, you have a layover in Berlin.*
- How long is the layover? *About 1 hour.*
- Do I have to change planes? *Yes, you have to change planes at …*
- How much carry-on luggage am I allowed?
- What weight am I allowed?
- My luggage is overweight. How much more do I need to pay?
- Is a meal served? *Yes, lunch will be served during the flight.*
- What time does the plane to Boston leave?
- When does the next flight to Boston leave?
- Can I get onto the next flight?
- Can I change my flight schedule?
- What's the departure time?
- Is the plane on time?
- What's the arrival time?
- Will I be able to make my connection?
- I have misplaced my hand luggage. Where is Lost Property?
- How much is it to upgrade this ticket to first class?
- I want to change the return flight date from Atlanta to Madrid to September 28th.
- Is it possible to purchase an open ticket?
- I have missed my flight to New York. When does the next flight leave, please?
- Can I use the ticket I have, or do I need to pay for a new one?

Announcing Changes in an Airline Flight

- *Our flight to Vigo has been canceled because of snow.*
- *Our flight to Chicago has been delayed; however, all connecting flights can be made.*
- *Flight number 0112 to Paris has been canceled.*
- *Flight number 1145 has been moved to gate B15.*
- *Passengers for flight number 110 to London, please proceed to gate 7. Hurry up!* Our flight has been called over the loudspeaker.

At the Boarding Gate

- *We will begin boarding soon.*
- *We are now boarding passengers in rows 24 through 36.*
- *May I see your boarding card?*

Arrival

- *Pick up your luggage at the terminal.*
- Where can I find a luggage cart?
- Where is the taxi rank?
- Where is the subway stop?
- Where is the way out?

Complaining about Lost or Damaged Luggage

- My luggage is missing.
- One of my bags seems to be missing.
- My luggage is damaged.
- One of my suitcases has been lost.

Exchange Office

- Where is the Exchange Office?
- What is the rate for the Dollar?
- Could you change 1000 Euros into Dollars?

Customs and Immigration Control

- *May I see your passport, please?*
- *Do you have your visa?*
- *What is your nationality?*
- *What is the purpose of your journey?* The purpose of my journey is …
- *How long do you plan on staying?*
- *Empty your pockets and put your wallet, keys, mobile phone and coins on this tray.*
- *Remove any metallic objects you are carrying and put them on this tray.*
- *Open your laptop.*
- *Take off your shoes. Put them in this tray too.*

- *Do you have anything to declare?* No, I don't have anything to declare.
- *Do you have anything to declare?* No, I only have personal effects.
- *Do you have anything to declare?* Yes, I am a doctor and I'm carrying some surgical instruments.
- *Do you have anything to declare?* Yes, I have bought six bottles of whisky and four cartons of cigarettes in the duty-free shop.
- *How much currency are you bringing into the country?* I haven't got any foreign currency.
- *Open your bag, please.*
- *I need to examine the contents of your bag.*
- May I close my bag? *Sure.*
- *Please place your suitcases on the table.*
- *What do you have in these parcels?* Some presents for my wife and kid.
- How much duty do I have to pay?
- Where is the Exchange Office?

During the Flight

Very few exchanges are likely during a normal flight. If you are familiar with them, you will realize how fluency interferes positively with your mood. Conversely, if you need a pillow and are not able to ask for it, your self-confidence will shrink, your neck will hurt, and you will not ask for anything else during the flight. Do not let lack of fluency spoil an otherwise perfect flight.

- Is there an aisle/window seat free? (I asked for one at the check-in and they told me I should ask onboard just in case there had been a cancellation).
- *Excuse me, you are in my seat.* Oh! Sorry, I didn't notice.
- *Fasten your seat belt, please.*
- *Your life-jacket is under your seat.*
- *Smoking is not allowed during the flight.*
- Please would you bring me a blanket/pillow?
- Is there a business class seat free?
- Can I upgrade to first class on board?
- *Would you like a cup of tea/coffee/a glass of soda?* A glass of soda, please.
- *What would you prefer, chicken or beef/fish or meat?* Beef/fish please.
- Is there a vegetarian menu?
- Stewardess, I'm feeling bad. Do you have anything for flight-sickness? Could you bring me another sick-bag please?

- Stewardess, I have a headache. Do you have an aspirin?
- Stewardess, this gentleman is disturbing me.

In the Taxi (US Cab)

Think for a moment of taking a taxi in your city. How many sentences do you suppose would be exchanged in normal, and even extraordinary, conditions? I assure you that with fewer than two dozen sentences you will solve more than 90% of possible situations.

Asking Where to Get a Taxi

- Where is the nearest taxi rank?
- Where can I get a taxi?

Basic Instructions

- Hi, take me downtown/to the Sheraton Hotel, please.
- Please would you take me to the airport?
- *It is rush hour; I don't go to the airport.*
- *Sorry, I am not on duty.*
- *It will cost you double fare to leave the city.*
- I need to go to the Convention Center.
- *Which way do you want me to take you, via Fifth or Seventh Avenue?* Either one would be OK.
- Is there any surcharge to the airport?

Concerning Speed in a Taxi

- To downtown as quick as you can.
- *Are you in a hurry?* Yes, I'm in a hurry.
- I'm late; please hurry up!
- Slow down!
- Do you have to drive so fast? There is no need to hurry. I am not in a rush at all.

Asking to Stop and Wait

- Stop at number 112, please.
- Which side of the street?
- *Do you want me to drop you at the door?*
- Pull over; I'll be back in a minute.
- Please, wait here a minute.
- Stop here.

Concerning the Temperature in a Taxi

- Would you please wind your window up? It's a bit cold.
- Could you turn the heat up/down/on/off?
- Could you turn the air conditioning on/off?
- Is the air conditioning/heating on?

Payment

- How much is it?
- How much do I owe you?
- Is the tip included?
- Do you have change for a twenty/fifty (dollar bill)? *Sorry, I don't (have any change).*
- Keep the change.
- Would you give me a receipt?
- I need a receipt, please.
- I think that is too expensive.
- They have never charged me this before. Give me a receipt, please. I think I'll make a complaint.
- Can I pay by credit card? *Sure, swipe your card here.*

At the Hotel

Checking in

- *May I help you?*
- Hello, I have reserved a room under the name of Dr. Pichard.
- *For how many people?* Two, my wife and me.
- Do you need my ID?
- Do you need my credit card?
- *How long will you be staying?* We are staying for a week.
- *You will have to wait until your room is ready.*
- *Here is your key.*
- *Enjoy your stay.* Thank you.
- Is there anybody who can help me with my bags?
- *Do you need a bellhop?* Yes, please.
- *I'll have someone bring your luggage up.*

Preferences

- Can you double-check that we have a double room with a view of the beach/city ...?
- I would like a room at the front/at the rear.
- I would like the quietest room you have.
- I would like a non-smoking room.
- I would like a suite.
- How many beds? I want a double bed/a single bed.
- I asked for two single beds.
- I'd like a king-sized bed.
- I'd like a queen-sized bed.
- We will need a crib for the baby.
- Are all your rooms en suite? *Yes, all of our rooms have a bath or shower.*
- Is breakfast included?
- Does the hotel have parking? (British English: "car park")
- Do you have a parking lot/structure nearby? (British English: "car park")

The Stay

- Can you give me a wake-up call at seven each morning?
- There is no hot water. Would you please send someone to fix it?
- The TV is not working properly. Would you please send someone to fix it?
- The bathtub has no plug. Would you please send someone up with one?
- The people in the room next to mine are making a racket. Would you please tell them to keep it down?
- I want to change my room. It's too noisy.
- What time does breakfast start?
- How can I get to the city center?
- Can we change Euros into Dollars?
- Could you recommend a good restaurant near to the hotel?
- Could you recommend a good restaurant?
- Would you give me the number for room service?
- I will have a cheese omelet, a ham sandwich, and an orange juice.
- Are there vending machines available?
- Do you have a fax machine available?
- Do you serve meals?
- Is there a pool/restaurant ...?
- How do I get room service?
- Is there wireless/Internet connection?
- The sink is clogged.
- The toilet is running.
- The toilet is leaking.
- My toilet overflowed!
- The toilet doesn't flush.
- The bath is leaking.
- My bathroom is flooded.
- The bath faucets (British English: "taps") drip day and night.
- The water is rust-colored.
- The pipes are always banging.
- The water is too hot.
- The water is never hot enough.
- I don't have any hot water.

Checking Out

- How much is it?
- Do you accept credit cards?
- Can I pay in Dollars/Euros?
- I'd like a receipt please.
- What time is checkout? Checkout is at 11 a.m.
- I would like to check out.
- Is there a penalty for late checkout?
- Please, would you have my luggage brought down?
- Would you please call me a taxi?:
- How far is the nearest bus stop/subway station?

Complaints

- Excuse me; there is a mistake on the receipt.
- I have had only one breakfast.
- I thought breakfast was included.
- I have been in a single room.
- Have you got a complaints book?
- Please would you give me my car keys?
- Is there anybody here who can help me with my luggage?

Course Example

General Information

By way of example, let us review some general information concerning a course program, focusing on those terms that may not be known by beginners.

Language

The official language of the course will be English.

Dress Code

Formal dress is required for the Opening Ceremony and for the Social Dinner. Casual wear is acceptable for all other events and occasions (although formal dress is customary for lecturers).

Commercial Exhibition

Participants will have the opportunity to visit representatives from pharmaceutical, diagnostic and equipment companies, and publishers at their stands to discuss new developments and receive up-to-date product information.

Although most beginners don't talk to salespeople due to their lack of fluency in English, talking to salespeople in commercial stands is a good way to practice cardiological English and, by the same token, receive up-to-date information on drugs, equipment and devices you currently use, or will use in the future, at your institution.

Disclosure Statements

To avoid commercial bias, speakers have to report whether they have significant relationships with industry or not.

As far as commercial relationships with industry are concerned, there are three types of speakers:
1. Speakers (spouses/partners, and planners) who have not reported significant relationships with industry.
2. Speakers who have reported receiving something of "value" from a company shoes product is related to the content of their presentations.
3. Speakers who have not provided information about their relationships with industry.

Faculty

Name and current posts of the speakers:

> • *Emilio R. Giuliani, M.D., Chair, Division of Cardiovascular Diseases, Mayo Clinic Scottsdale, Scottsdale, Arizona*

"Guest Faculty" includes those speakers coming from institutions other than those organizing the course.

How to Reach ...

Arrival by plane
The international airport is situated about 25 kilometers outside the city. To reach the city center you can use the:

> • *City airport train. Every half-hour. Non-stop. 18 minutes from the airport direct to downtown, and from downtown direct to the airport. Fare: single, EUR 10; return, EUR 18.*

- *Regional railway, line 6. Travel time: 36 minutes. Frequency: every 30 minutes. Fare: Single, EUR 12; Return EUR 20. Get off at "Charles Square." From there use the underground line "U7" to "Park Street."*
- *Bus. International Airport to … Charles Square. Travel time: 25 minutes. Fare: EUR 8.*
- *Taxi. There is a taxi rank to the south of the arrival hall. A taxi to the city center costs around EUR 45 (depending on traffic).*

Arrival by train
For detailed information about the timetable you can call …

At the railway station you can use the underground to reach the city.

Congress venue (where the course is to be held, e.g., hotel, university, convention center …):

Continental Hotel
32 Park Street, 23089 …
Phone: …/Fax: …
E-mail: continentalhotel@hhs.com

To reach the venue from the city center (Charles Square) take the U1 underground line (green). Leave the train at Park Street and take the exit marked Continental Hotel. Traveling time: approximately 10 minutes.

Financial Matters

The common European currency is the Euro.

Weather

The weather in … in December is usually cold with occasional snow. The daytime temperatures normally range from –5 to +5 °C.

Registration

Generally you will have been registered beforehand and you will not have to register at the course's registration counter. If you do have to register at the congress venue, then the following are some of the most usual exchanges that may take place during registration:

Cardiologist: May I have a registration form, please?

Course attendant: *Do you want me to fill it out (UK fill it in) for you?*
                     Are you a cardiologist?
                     Are you an ESC member?
                     Are you attending the full course?

Cardiology resident:	No. I'm a cardiology resident.
Course attendant:	*Can I see your chairperson's confirmation letter?*
Cardiology resident:	I was told it was faxed last week. Would you check that, please?
Cardiologist:	I'll pay by cash/credit card. Charge it to my credit card. Would you make out an invoice?
Course attendant:	*Do you need an invoice?* *Do you want me to draw up an invoice?*
Cardiologist:	Where should I get my badge?
Course attendant:	*Join that line.*

Course Planning

The basic idea whenever you attend an international cardiology course is that you must rehearse beforehand those situations that are inevitably going to happen and, in so doing, you will keep to a minimum embarrassing situations catching you off-guard. If only I had rehearsed (at home!) the meaning of the word "badge," I would not have been caught by surprise on my first course abroad. Just a few words, set phrases, and collocations must be known in a cardiological course environment, and we can assure you that knowing them will give you the confidence needed to make your participation in the course a personal success.

The first piece of advice is: *Read the program of the course thoroughly and look up in the dictionary or ask your more experience colleagues about the words and concepts you don't know. Since the program is available before the course starts, go over it at home; you don't need to read the scientific program at the course's venue.*

"Adjourn" is one of those typical program terms with which one gets familiar once the session is "adjourned." Although many could think that most terms are going to be integrated and understood by their context, our intention is to go over those "insignificant" terms that may prevent you from optimizing your time at the course.

The course plan may contain the following elements:

- *Main sessions* are sessions in which renowned experts present state-of-the-art reviews on clinical cardiology, basic and clinical cardiovascular research, and epidemiology, with a perspective for today's clinical practice.
- *Symposia* allow for in-depth discussion of recent developments in the various fields of basic science, epidemiology, and clinical cardiology.

- *Debates* provide a lively yet balanced discussion on controversial issues.
- *How-to sessions* give a unique opportunity for intense interaction between a limited audience and two or three experts in various fields of clinical cardiology.
- *Clinical seminars* are designed to highlight what every clinician should know about specific subspecialty topics.
- *Basic science track* is a series of sessions focusing on basic science related to cardiovascular disease. Renowned scientists review vascular biology, muscle biology, molecular biology, and other areas of basic science related to the physiology and pathophysiology of the cardiovascular system. These sessions will be particularly attractive for basic scientists, but also for clinicians with an interest in basic science.
- *Meet the experts* are one-hour lunch-time sessions that focus on practical management of cardiovascular diseases in daily situations. Each session deals with two case presentations discussed by a panel of experts, and refer to current ESC guidelines.
- *Read with the experts.* Don't miss these discussions around practical cases, by experts who will be able to explain difficulties, pitfalls and limitations of these new techniques. These sessions will take place during the coffee breaks.
- *Science hot line.* This session allows for submission of late-breaking experimental work.
- *Bench-to-bedside* sessions presenting new science with emerging clinical implications dedicated to basic scientists as well as clinicians.
- *FOCUS cardiology practice.* These sessions address the needs of practicing cardiologists, focusing on patient-oriented clinical decision-making. Experienced clinicians will present cases and discuss diagnostic and therapeutic options with the audience in an interactive manner. The application of guidelines and optimal patient management, based on clinical observations, laboratory examinations, echocardiography, electrophysiology, angiography, and other investigations are critically reviewed.
- *FOCUS imaging intervention.* The FOCUS imaging intervention sessions address current problems and new developments in catheter-based and surgical interventions, as well as non-invasive diagnostic procedures. Experts will demonstrate these techniques live, and a panel will discuss their indications and their use in daily patient care. These sessions integrate unlimited audiovisual facilities, and interaction with the audience will be stimulated using a voting system.

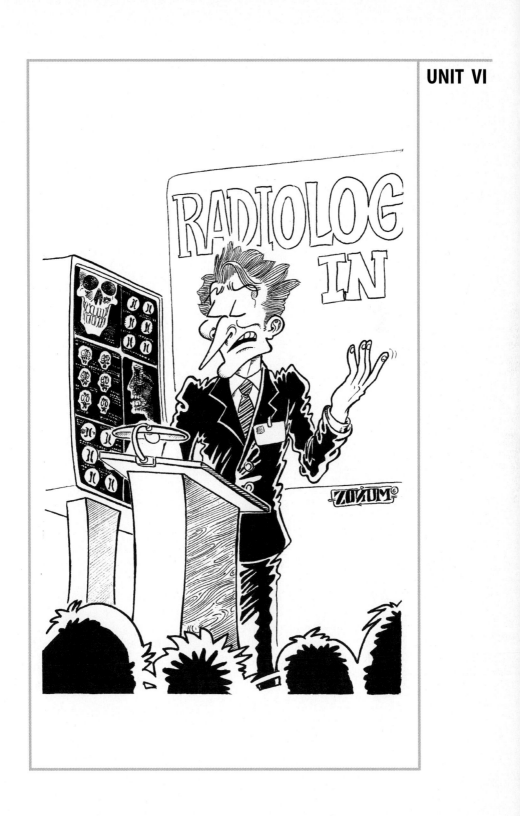

Unit VI Giving a Cardiological Talk

Introduction

International cardiological conferences are in a universe of their own. In this universe, attendees and speakers come from many different countries, with their own cultures and consequently, their own habits in terms of behavior and public speaking. However, most speakers set aside, at least partially, their cultural identity to embrace the international medical conference style. This standardization is part of the globalization that we are all witnessing.

The most widely spoken language is not Chinese, English or Spanish anymore, but the new phenomenon of broken English. This language is the result of simplifying English to make it as neutral and understandable as possible, removing colloquial idioms, regional expressions or any other source of linguistic confusion.

In this new universe, health-care professionals find themselves having to make a conscious effort to adapt to these explicit and implicit rules. Some of them are discussed in the following sections.

Having read this chapter, you will not only be able to improve your presentations or feel at ease giving them, but you might also actually end up being able to convey your message and who knows? You might even enjoy it – even if you have to deliver your presentation in the graveyard slot (the "graveyard slot" is the first presentation after lunch when most of the audience will be suffering from postprandial somnolence and very likely you will not hear a sound except for snores).

Dos and Don'ts

Time is also a very cultural thing. This peculiarity should be taken into account. Eight o'clock in the morning might seem an early start in Latin America but a perfectly normal starting time in northern Europe and the United States. Furthermore, the day is divided differently in various parts of the world ... and in our cardiological universe. Thus at an international conference the day is divided into:

- The morning: from the start time to noon
- The afternoon: from 12:01 to 17:00 or 18:00
- The evening: from 18:00 to midnight
- *Do* remember to follow these tips:
  - *Good morning:* from the start time to 12:00
  - *Good afternoon:* from 12:01 onward, even though your metabolism is far from feeling afternoon-ish until your usual lunch time has gone by and is begging you to say "good morning"
  - *Good evening:* from 18:00 onward. Note that if we have to give a presentation, make a speech or offer a toast at 22:00, we should never begin with "good night"; that should be reserved only for when we are going to bed. So "good night" is not supposed to be said in public.

When giving a presentation, there is always a time limit. I understand, and have actually experienced myself, how difficult it is to cram all we have to say about the topic that we have been researching over the last few years into a mere 20 min. In view of this time constraint, there are various alternatives ranging from speaking as fast as the tongue can rattle, to cutting it down to 5 min and spending the other 15 min vacantly gazing at the audience. American, British, and Australian physicians are often extremely fluent speakers (we know, we know ... they are using their mother tongue). However, remember that showing and commenting on five slides a minute and speaking faster than can be registered on a digital recorder might not be the best way to conveying a message.

- *Don't* speak too fast or too slowly.
- *Don't* say "sorry for this slide." Since you are the one who chooses the slides to be presented, get rid of those you would have to apologize for.
- *Do* summarize your presentation and rehearse to see how long you need for a clear delivery.

Sometimes lecturers tend to give too much data and minor details in their presentations. Their introduction is often full of information that is of little relevance to the international audience (for example, the name, date and code of local, provincial, regional and national laws regulating cardiological standards in his/her institution, or even the background information on the main researchers of a trial, including their graduation year and shoe size ... or a full history of the sixteenth-century building where the hospital stands today and subsequent restorations it has undergone, etc.). In these cases, by the time all these details have been given and the presentation has passed the introduction stage, time is up and the chairperson starts making desperate signs to the speaker.

- *Do* grab the pointer with both hands.

The best way of avoiding a trembling pointer is to grab it with both hands and place them over the lectern. If this does not work, we recommend using the mouse since, at least, your trembling will be confined to one plane instead of the three-dimensional shaking of a laser pointer.

- *Do* use either a pointer or the computer's mouse.

Although it may seem unbelievable, I attended a lecture in which the presenter, instead of using a laser pointer, directed the audience's attention to the images using a folded newspaper. The only person who could see the details the speaker was pointing out was the speaker himself.

- *Do* structure your presentation so that you convey a few clear messages instead of a huge amount of not-so-relevant information that nobody has a chance to take in.
- *Don't* read slides, but instead try to explain a few basic ideas as clearly as possible.

Many intermediate-English-speaking doctors could not agree with this point because they can only feel some confidence if they read the presentation. Reading is the least-natural means of communicating experiences; we encourage you to present your paper without reading it. Although it will need much more intensive preparation, the delivery will be more fluid and – why not? – even brilliant. Many foreign doctors resign themselves to delivering just acceptable talks and explicitly reject the possibility of making a presentation at the same level as they would in their own language. Do not reject the possibility of being as brilliant as you would be in your own language; the only difference is in the amount of rehearsal. Thorough rehearsal can provide you with amazing results; do not give up beforehand.

- *Don't* read your presentation from a script.

Even worse than reading slides is to read from a script. I have witnessed complete messes happening to lecturers who tried, without any success at all, to coordinate scribbled pages on the lectern and slides. The noise of the passing pages was unbearable and the face of a speaker on the verge of a mental breakdown kept the audience from listening to the presentation itself.

- *Do* enjoy yourself.

When giving the presentation, relax; nobody knows more than you do about the specific subject that you are presenting. The only way to make people enjoy your presentation is by enjoying it yourself. You only have to communicate, not to perform; being a good researcher or a competent clinician is not the same thing as being a stand-up comedian or a model. This does not mean that we can afford to overlook our presentation skills, especially if you want most of your colleagues to still be awake at the end of your presentation!

- *Do* try to overcome stage fright and focus on communicating.

There must be somebody out there interested in what you have to say ... either to praise it or to tear it to pieces, but that does not matter.

- *Do* avoid anything that would make you nervous when giving your presentation.

One piece of advice is to remove all keys, coins, or other metal objects from your pockets so that you are not tempted to rattle them around – a truly irritating noise that we have all learned to hate.

- *Do* put your cell (UK: mobile) phone and beeper on "Silent."

The only thing more embarrassing than an attendee's cell phone interrupting your lecture is your own phone ringing in the middle of your talk.

- *Do* make sure that your jokes can be understood internationally.

Creativity and humor are always appreciated in a lecture hall, providing they are both appropriate and understood! We all know that humor is a very cultural thing, like time-keeping, ties, food preferences, etc. Almost all American speakers will start their presentation with a joke that most Europeans will not understand, not even the Irish or British. A British speaker will probably throw in the most sarcastic comment when you are least expecting it and in the same tone as if he or she were telling you about the mortality rate in his or her unit. A foreign (neither American nor British) doctor might just try to tell a long joke in English based on a play on words in his or her mother tongue which obviously doesn't work in English, and possibly involves religion, sport and/or sex (as a general rule avoid religious and sex jokes in public presentations).

Useful Sentences for Cardiological Talks

Introducing the Presentation

- Good afternoon. It is an honor to have the opportunity to speak to you about ...
- Good afternoon. Thank you for your kind introduction. It is my pleasure to speak to you about an area of great interest to me.
- In the next few minutes I'll talk about ...
- The topic I'll cover this afternoon is ...
- In the next 20 minutes I'll show you ...
- In my talk on diastolic function, I want to share with you all our experience on ...

- Thank you for sticking around (informal way of addressing the last talk attendees).
- I'd like to thank you Dr. Leon for his kind invitation.
- Thank you Dr. Pichard for inviting me to attend this course.
- Thank you Dr. Nieminen. It is a great honor to be here talking about ...
- On behalf of my colleagues and assistants, I want to thank Dr. Palacios for his kind invitation.
- I'd like to welcome you to this course on ...(to be said in the first talk of the course if you are a member of the organizing committee).
- Today, I want to talk to you about ...
- Now, allow me to introduce ...
- What I want to talk about this morning is ...
- During the next few minutes, I'd like to draw your attention to ...
- First of all, let me summarize the contents of my lecture on ...
- Let's begin by looking at these 3D images of the heart ...

Commenting on Images, Graphs, Tables, Schematic Representations, Etc

- As you can see in the image on your right ...
- As you will see in the next table ...
- As we saw in the previous slide ...
- The next image shows ...
- The next image allows us to ...
- In the bottom left image we can see ...
- What do we have to look at here?
- What do we have to bear in mind with regard to this artifact?
- Notice how the lesion is ...
- Bear in mind that this image was obtained in less than 10 seconds ...
- Let's look at this schematic representation of the mitral valve.
- As you can see in this CT image ...
- Let us have a look at this schematic diagram of the mitral valve.
- Looking at this table, you can see ...
- Having a look at this bar chart, we could conclude that ...
- To sum up, let's look at this diagram ...
- The image on your right ...
- The image at the top of the screen shows ...
- Let's turn to the next slide in which the lesion, after balloon dilatation, becomes clearly irregular.
- Figure 3 brings out the importance of ...
- As can be observed in this MR image ...

- I apologize that the faint area of sclerosis in the aortic valve *does not project well*. (When a subtle finding is difficult to see on a projected image, it is said that *it does not project well*.)
- On the left of the screen is an IVUS image at the level of the deployed stent. On the right of the screen there is another image, showing complete apposition of stent's struts after complete expansion.

Summing Up

- To sum up we can say that ...
- In summary, we have discussed ...
- To conclude ...
- Summing up, I would say that ...
- The take-home lesson of the talk is ...
- To put it in a nutshell ...
- To cut a long story short ...
- In short, ...
- To put it briefly ...
- Be that as it may, we have to bear in mind that ...
- If there is one point I hope you will take away from this presentation, it is that ...
- CT has proven to be very useful in the non-invasive assessment of coronary arteries by providing additional information during image interpretation.
- Cardiac MRI is a powerful technique that yields valuable diagnostic information.
- The rate of growth and distribution of cardiac CT will depend on investing in technology, training and collaboration.
- MRI may be helpful in the management of ... if sonography is inconclusive.
- Virtual angiography is the most modern technique for the assessment of ...

Concluding

- Thank you for your kind attention.
- Thank you all for sticking around until the very last talk of the session.
- Thank you all.
- Thank you very much for your time; you have been a most gracious audience.

- Thank you for your attention. I would be happy to entertain any questions.
- Thank you for your time. I would be happy to address any questions.
- This is all we have time for, so thank you, and have a good time in London.
- Let me finish my presentation by saying that ...
- We can say to conclude that ...
- Let me end by wishing you a pleasant stay in our city.
- I'd be happy to answer any question you might have.
- I'd be happy to address your comments and questions.
- Ignore lesions less than 4 mm in your reports.

The Dreaded Questions-and-Comments Section

Many beginners would not hesitate to deliver a free communication at an international congress if there were not a short section of questions after them.

This anecdote may illustrate the feelings of many non–native English-speaking cardiologists in their first presentation in English.

After a short free communication on the MR follow-up of a Ross operation (the surgical replacement of a patient's aortic valve by the pulmonary valve and the replacement of the latter by a homograft), which had so far gone reasonably well for a beginner, I was waiting, like a rabbit staring at a snake, for the round of questions that inevitably followed my presentation.

On the very verge of a mental breakdown, I listened to an English radiologist asking me a question I could barely understand. I asked him, "Would you please repeat your question?" and he, obediently, repeated the question with exactly the same words and the same pace with which he had formulated it before. As I could not understand the question the second time, the chairperson roughly translated it into a more international and easily understandable English and I finally answered it. This was the only question I was asked since the time was over and there was no room for any other comment.

Let us think about this anecdote in a positive way by dissecting it into the following points, which will lead us to some recommendations.

1. Do not be discouraged. Nobody told you that beginnings were easy.
2. Questions and comments by native English speakers tend to be more difficult to understand.
3. There are several types of interlocutors of which you must be aware.
4. Do not complain if the interlocutor does exactly what you asked him/her for.

5. Chairmen can always help you.
6. Time is limited and you can take advantage of this fact.

These points lead to some recommendations:

1. I did not know by then that the worst was still to come. I wasted the whole morning recreating the scene over and over. "How could I have wasted so many hours of research and study? I even thought that people recognized me as the one who didn't understand a simple query ..." Let us think for a moment how you performed the first time you did anything in your life, i.e., the first time you grabbed a tennis racquet or a golf club. In comparison to that, it was not that bad.

2. When the cardiologist who asked for the microphone is a non–native English speaker you can begin to feel better since you are going to talk to an equal with regard to language, to one who has spent a great number of hours fighting to learn a language other than his/her own. On the other hand, when you have to deal with a native English speaker, there are two main types of interlocutors.
   - *Type A* is a colleague who does not take advantage of being a native English speaker and reduces his/her normal rhythm of speech so you can understand the question and, therefore, convey to the audience whatever you have to say.
   - *Type B* is a colleague who does not make any allowance for the difference between native and non–native English lecturers. Needless to say, I faced a type B interlocutor in my first international presentation.

3. Types of interlocutors:
   a. *Type 1*. The interlocutor who wants to know a particular detail of your presentation. These interlocutors are easy to handle by just answering their question.
      i. Question: *What diameters do you measure in the aortic root?*
      ii. Answer: Annulus, Valsalva sinuses, and sinotubular junction.
   b. *Type 2*. The interlocutor who wants the audience to notice his sound knowledge of the subject which is being discussed. These interlocutors are quite easy to handle as well since they do not formulate questions as such but make a point of their own. The replies tend to be shorter than the questions/comments and time, which runs in favor of the beginner provided he is not speaking, goes by, leaving no room for another dreadful question.
      i. *I do agree with your comments.*
      ii. *We are planning to include this point in our next paper on ...*
   c. Type 3. The interlocutor who strongly disagrees with your points. This is obviously the most difficult to handle for a beginner due to the scarcity of his idiomatic resources. The only piece of advice is none other than that you must defend your points from a humble position, and do not ever challenge your interlocutor.

    i. I will consider your suggestions on …

    ii. This is a work in progress and we will consider including your suggestions …

4. If I had requested my interlocutor to ask his question again more slowly and in a different way so I could understand it, then he would have been morally obliged to do so. But beginners lack this kind of modesty and pretend to be better and know more than they actually are and do, which is, by definition, a mistake. Better is, "I don't understand your question. Would you please reformulate your question in a different way, please?"

5. When you feel you need some help, ask the chairperson to help you out: "Dr. Ramee (chairperson), I'm not sure I've understood the question. Would you please formulate it in a different way?"

6. It is, at worst, 1 min of stress. Do not let such a short period of time prevent you from a potentially successful career in international cardiology.

Sentences That May Help

Go over these sentences; they may help you escape from a difficult situation and minimize your fear of questions and comments section:

Making Your Point

- Let me point out that murmur intensity is paramount in order to differentiate …
- You must bear in mind that this 3D reconstruction was obtained …
- If you look closely at this atrial septal defect, then you will realize …
- I want to draw your attention to the fact that …
- Don't forget the importance of anticoagulation in …
- Before I move on to my next slide …
- In view of the upcoming publication of …
- From a cardiological point of view …
- As far as trackability is concerned …
- The bottom line of the subject is …

Giving Explanations

- To put it in another way, chemical shift artifact was responsible for ...
- Taking into consideration that the cardioversion was done under conscious sedation ...
- In a bit more detail, you can notice that ...
- This fact can be explained taking into account that ...
- EKG tracing was poor since the patient could not hold his breath.
- Although double antiplatelet regime was well tolerated by most patients ...
- In short, you may need larger balloons in Scandinavian patients.
- What I'm saying is that sudden death is related to abnormal growth of myocardial tissue.
- We did not administer pain killers because the patient refused it.
- We performed a normal echocardiography because the patient suffered from esophageal stenosis.

Answering Multiple Questions

- There are two different questions here.
- It seems there are three questions here.
- It is my understanding that there are two questions to be addressed here.
- Regarding your second question, ...
- As far as your first question is concerned, ...
- Answering your first question, I should say that ...
- I'll begin with your second question.
- Let me address your last question first.
- I'll address your last question first and then the rest of them.
- Would you please repeat your second question?
- I didn't understand your first question. Would you repeat it?

Disagreeing

- With all due respect, I believe that there is no evidence of ...
- To the best of our knowledge no article has been published on this topic.
- With all respect, I think that your point overlooks the main aspect of ...
- Yours is an interesting point of view, but I'm not sure of its ...
- I see it from a different point of view.
- With all respect, I don't go along with you on ...
- I think that the importance of ... cannot be denied.
- I strongly disagree with your comment on ...

- I disagree with your point.
- I don't see a valid argument for supporting such a comment.

Emphasizing a Point

- I do believe that ...
- I strongly agree with Dr. Garland's comment on ...
- It is of paramount importance ...
- It is a crucial fact that ...
- And this fact cannot be overlooked.
- I'd like to stress the importance of ...
- Don't underestimate the role of ...
- The use of Flecainide in this case is of the utmost importance.
- With regard to ..., you must always bear in mind that ...
- It is well known that ...

Incomprehension

- I'm not sure I understood your question ...
- Sorry, I don't quite follow you.
- Would you repeat the question, please?
- Would you repeat the second part of your question, please?
- I'm afraid I still don't understand.
- Could you be a bit more specific with regard to ...?
- What do you mean by ...?
- Could you repeat your question? I couldn't hear you.
- Could you formulate your question in a different way?
- I'm not sure I understand your final question.

Playing for Time

- I am not sure I understood your question. Would you repeat it?
- I don't understand your questions. Would you formulate it in a different way?
- That's a very interesting question ...
- I wonder if you could be a bit more specific about ...
- I'm glad you asked that question.
- Your question is of the utmost importance, but I'm afraid it is beyond the scope of our paper ...
- What aspect of the problem are you referring to by saying ...

Evading an Issue

- I'm afraid I'm not really in a position to be able to address your question yet.
- We'll come back to that in a minute, if you don't mind.
- I don't think we have enough time to discuss your comments in depth.
- It would take extremely long time to answer that.
- I will address your question in my second talk, if you don't mind.
- At my institution, we do not have experience on ...
- At our department, we do not perform ...
- Perhaps we could return to that at the end of the session.
- We'll probably address your question in further papers on the subject.
- I have no experience. ...

Technical Problems

- May I have another laser pointer?
- Does anyone in the audience have a pointer?
- Video images are not running properly. In the meantime I'd like to comment on ...
- My microphone is not working properly. May I have it fixed?
- My microphone is not working properly. May I use yours?
- Can you hear me?
- Can the rows at the back hear me?
- Can you guys at the back see the screen?
- Can we turn of the lights please?

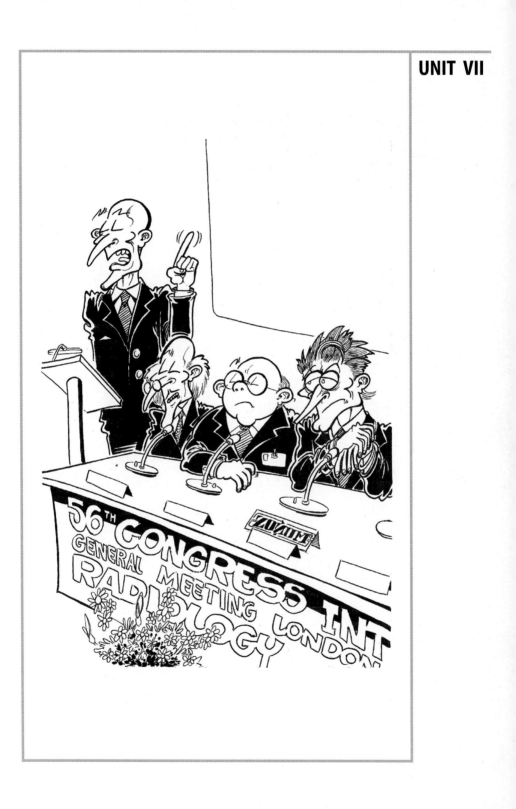

Unit VII   Chairing a Cardiovascular Session

Introduction

Chairing sessions at international meetings usually comes up when you have reached a certain level in your academic career. To reach this point, many papers will have been submitted and many presentations will have been given, so the chances are your level of medical English will be above that of the target audience of this manual.

The reason to include this chapter – contrary to what many of those who have never chaired a session in an international meeting may think – even an experienced chairperson may face difficult, even embarrassing situations.

For those who have never chaired a session, to be a chairperson means, first, not having to prepare a presentation, and, second, the use of simple sentences such as "thank you Dr. Smith, for your interesting presentation" or "the next speaker will be Dr. Spurek who comes from …".

In our opinion, being a chairperson means much more than one who has never chaired them might think. To begin with, a chairperson must go over not one presentation, but thoroughly study all the recently published material on the subject under discussion. On top of that, a chairperson must review all the abstracts and must have prepared questions just in case the audience has no questions or comments.

We have divided this section into four subsections:

1. Usual chairperson's comments
2. Should chairpersons ask questions?
3. What the chairperson should say when something is going wrong
4. Specific cardiological chairperson's comments.

Usual Chairperson's Comments

Everybody who has attended an international meeting is aware of the usual sentences the chairperson uses to introduce the session. Certain key expressions will provide you with a sense of fluency, without which chairing a session would be troublesome. The good news is that if you know the key sentences and use them appropriately, then chairing a session is easy. The bad news is that if, on the contrary, you do not know these expressions, then a theoretically simple task will become an embarrassing situation. There is always a first time for everything, and if it is the first time you have been invited to chair a session, rehearse some of these sentences and you will feel quite comfortable. Accept this piece of advice: Only "rehearsed spontaneity" looks spontaneous if you are a beginner.

Introducing the Session

We suggest the following useful comments for introducing speakers:

- Our first speaker is Dr. Spurek from Xanit International Hospital in Málaga, Spain, who will present the paper "Left Ventricular Diastolic Filling Pattern in Patients with Dilated Cardiomyopathy."

The following speakers are introduced almost the same way with sentences such as:

- Our next lecturer is Dr. Ashy. Dr. Ashy comes from Brigham and Women's Hospital, Harvard Medical School, and his presentation is entitled "Primary Angioplasty Using DES."
- Next is Dr. Shaw from Beth Israel Deaconess Hospital, presenting "Door-to-Needle Time in Non-Anterior Myocardial Infarction. Long-Term Follow-Up."
- Dr. Barba from University Clinic of Navarre is the next and last speaker. His presentation is "Role of Echocardiography in Acute Myocardial Infarction."

Once the speakers finish their presentation, the chairperson is supposed to say something like:

- Thank you, Dr. Barba, for your excellent presentation. Any questions or comments?

The chairperson usually comments on presentations, although sometimes they do not:

- Thank you, Dr. Barba, for your presentation. Any questions or comments from the audience?

There are some common adjectives (*nice, elegant, outstanding, excellent, interesting, clear, accurate*) and formulas that are usually used to describe presentations. These are illustrated in the following comments:

- Thanks, Dr. Shaw, for your accurate presentation. Does the audience have any comments?
- Thank you very much for your clear presentation on this always-controversial topic. I would like to ask a question. May I? (Although being the chairperson you are the one who gives permission, to ask the speaker is a usual formality.)
- I'd like to thank you for this excellent talk Dr. Olsen. Any questions?
- Thanks a lot for your talk, Dr. Barba. I wonder if the audience has any questions.

Adjourning

We suggest the following useful comments for adjourning the session:

- I think we all are a bit tired, so we'll have a short break.
- The session is adjourned until 4 p.m.
- We'll take a short break.
- We'll take a 30-minute break. Please fill out the evaluation forms.
- The session is adjourned until tomorrow morning. Enjoy your stay in Paris.

Finishing the Session

We suggest the following useful comments for finishing the session:

- I'd like to thank all the speakers and the audience for your interesting presentations and comments. (I'll) see you all at the congress dinner and awards ceremony.
- The session is over. I want to thank all the participants for their contribution. (I'll) see you tomorrow morning. Remember to take your attendance certificates if you have not taken them already.
- We should finish up over here. We'll resume at 10.50.

Should Chairpersons Ask Questions?

In our opinion, chairpersons are supposed to ask questions, especially at the beginning of the session when the audience does not usually make any comments at all. Warming-up the session is one of the chairperson's duties, and if nobody in the audience is in the mood to ask questions the chairperson must invite the audience to participate:

- Are there any questions?

Nobody raises a hand:

- Well, I have two questions for Dr. Viola. Do you think IVUS is the method of choice for the detection of coronary vulnerable plaques? Second, what should be, in your opinion, the role of multislice CT in this diagnostic algorithm?

Once the session has been warmed-up, the chairperson should only ask questions or add comments as a tool to manage the timing of the session, so that, as is usual, the session is behind schedule, the chairperson is not required to participate unless strictly necessary.

The chairperson does not have to demonstrate to the audience his or her knowledge on the discussed topics by asking too many questions or making comments. The chairperson's knowledge of the subject is not in doubt since without it, he or she would not have been selected to chair.

What the Chairperson Should Say When Something Is Going Wrong

Behind Schedule

Many lecturers, knowing beforehand they have a certain amount of time to deliver their presentations, try to talk a little bit more, stealing time from the questions/comments time and from later speakers. Chairpersons should cut short this tendency at the very first chance:

- Dr. Cutty, your time is almost over. You have 30 seconds to finish your presentation.
- Dr. Shang, you are running out of time.

If the speaker does not finish his presentation on time, the chairperson may say:

- Dr. Cutty, I'm sorry but your time is over. We must proceed to the next presentation. Any questions, comments?

After introducing the next speaker, sentences such as the following will help you handle the session:

- Dr. Treasure, please keep an eye on the time, we are behind schedule.
- We are far from being ahead of schedule, so I remind all speakers you have 6 minutes to deliver your presentation.

Ahead of Schedule

Although unusual, sometimes there is some extra time and this is a good chance to ask the panelists a general question about their experience at their respective institutions:

- As we are a little bit ahead of schedule, I encourage the panelists and the audience to ask questions and offer comments.
- I have a question for the panelists: What percentage of the total number of coronary angiograms is performed on women?

Technical Problems

Computer Not Working

We suggest the following comments:

- I am afraid there is a technical problem with the computer. In the meantime I would like to make a comment about ...
- The computer is not working properly. While it is being fixed, I encourage the panelists to offer their always-interesting comments.

Lights Have Gone Out

We suggest the following comments:

- The lights have gone out. We'll take a (hopefully) short break until they are repaired.
- As you see, or indeed do not see at all, the lights have gone out. The hotel staff has told us it is going to be a matter of minutes, so do not go too far; we'll resume as soon as possible.

Sound Has Gone Off

We suggest the following comments:

- Dr. Kannel, we cannot hear you. There must be a problem with your microphone.
- Perhaps you could try this microphone.
- Please would you use the microphone? The rows at the back cannot hear you.

Lecturer Lacks Confidence

If the lecturer is speaking too quietly:

- Dr. Ramee, would you please speak up? The audience cannot hear you.
- Dr. Barba, would you please speak up a bit? The people at the back cannot hear you.

If the lecturer is so nervous he/she cannot go on delivering the presentation:

- Dr. Garcia, take your time. We can proceed to the next presentation, so whenever you feel OK and ready to deliver yours, it will be a pleasure to listen to it.

Specific Cardiological Chairperson's Comments

Since the chairpersons are supposed to fill in the gaps in the session, if a technical problem occurs, then the chairperson must say something "to entertain" the audience in the meantime. This fact would not create any problem to a native English speaker but may be troublesome for a non-native English speaking chairperson. In these situations, there is an always-helpful topic to be addressed "in the meantime," namely, the current situation of what is discussed in the session in the panelists' countries.

- Regarding OCT, how are things going in Italy, Dr. Novo?
- As for the use of Amplatzer closure device, what's the ideal in Japan, Dr. Nakamura?
- How is the current situation in Germany regarding repayment policies?
- May I ask how many coronary angiograms you are performing yearly at your respective institutions?
- What's going on in the States, Dr. Leon?

By opening a discussion on how things are going in different countries, the not-too-fluent chairperson shares the burden of filling in the gaps with the panelists. This trick rarely fails, and once the technical problem is fixed, the session can go on normally with nobody in the audience noticing the lack of fluency of the chairperson.

Besides the usual expressions chairpersons of whatever medical specialty have to be aware of, there are typical comments a cardiologic chairperson should be familiar with. These comments vary, depending on the cardiologic subspecialty of the chairperson and are, generally speaking, easy to deal with for even non-native English speakers. By way of example, let us review the following:

- Dr. Lucas, would you please use the pointer so the audience knows what lesion you are talking about?
- Dr. Wilson, would you please point out the defect area so we can distinguish the ischemic myocardium from the normal one?
- Dr. Crisóstomo, did you perform a coronary CT scan on this patient?
- Dr. Maier, did you perform the 2D-echo on an emergent basis?
- Dr. Olsen, I can't see the lesion you are talking about. Can you point it out?
- Have you had any adverse anaphylactic reactions to this type of contrast material?
- Do you use 5F catheters for this purpose?
- Dr. Castañeda, I'm afraid that the video is not running properly. Could you try to fix it so we can see your excellent cardiac MR images?
- Dr. Nakamura, why didn't you use a lower profile balloon to cross the stenosis?
- Dr. Mesa, are you currently using dobutamine in cases like this one?
- Dr. Fernandez, is trackability that important in these cases?
- Dr. Marco, do you use IVUS or OCT in every patient after the stent has been deployed?
- Do you routinely perform stress test to evaluate coronary stent follow-up?
- Dr. Benitez, why didn't you make primary angioplasty instead of thrombolysis on this young patient?

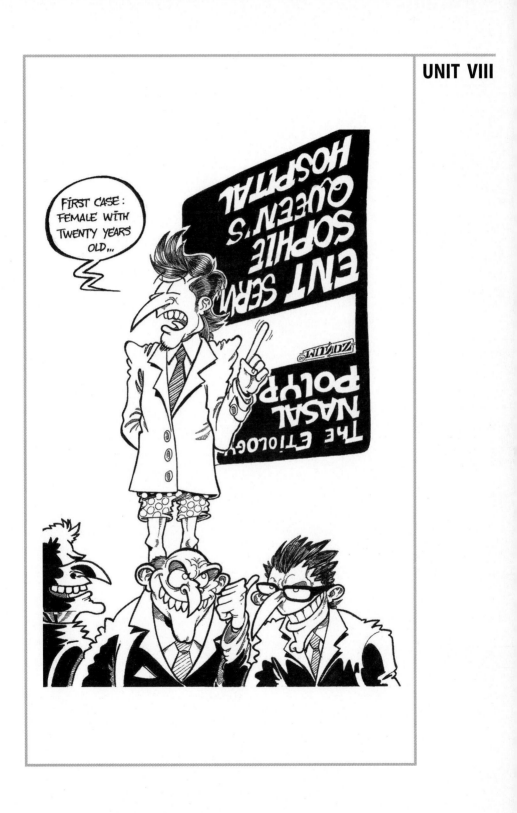

Unit VIII   Usual Mistakes Made by Cardiologists Speaking and Writing in English

Introduction

In this section, we try to share with you what we have found to be some of the great hurdles in cardiologic English. Many things certainly can go wrong when one is asked to give a lecture in English or whenever one is supposed to communicate in cardiologic English. This is by no means an exhaustive account; it is just a way of passing on what we have learnt from our own experience in the fascinating world of cardiologic English.

When preparing and actually delivering a presentation in English at an international cardiologic conference, a series of basic issues should be taken into account. We have grouped them into four danger zones, in the hope that their classification will make them become less of a problem. The categories are the following:

1. Misnomers and false friends
2. Common grammatical mistakes
3. Common spelling mistakes
4. Common pronunciation mistakes.

Misnomers and False Friends

Every tongue has its own false friends. A thorough review of false friends is beyond the scope of this manual, and we suggest that you look for those tricky names that sound similar in your language and in English but have completely different meanings.

Think, for example, about the term *graft-versus-host disease*. The translation of *host* has not been correct in some romance languages, and in Spanish the term *host*, which in this context means recipient, has been translated as *huésped*, which means *person staying in another's house*. Many Spanish medical students have problems with the understanding of this disease because of the terminology used. Taking into account that what actually happens is that the graft reacts against the recipient, if the disease had been named *graft-versus-recipient disease*, the concept would probably be more precisely conveyed.

So from now on, identify false friends in your own language and make a list beginning with those belonging to your specialty; it is no use knowing false friends in a language different from your own.

Medicine in general and Anatomy in particular are full of misnomers. Think for a moment about the term *superficial femoral vein*. It is difficult to explain how a superficial femoral vein clot is actually in the deep venous system.

Many radiologists, cardiologist and oncologists all over the world say *small (mediastinal) lymphadenopathies* when evaluating a thorax CT. Taking into account that size is the only criterion for the diagnosis of abnormal lymph nodes and that lymphadenopathy means, from an etymological point of view, *abnormal lymph node*, a "normal" (*small-size*) *lymphadenopathy* is as absurd as a *normal psychopathy*. The term *lymphadenomegaly* would probably be a more accurate one.

Etymologically, *azygos* means *odd*, which puts *hemiazygos* in a strange situation since odd numbers are not divisible by 2.

The term *innominate vein* is as absurd as naming a baby *unnamed*.

Common Grammatical Mistakes

1. The chairperson of cardiology came from an university hospital.

2. Although university starts with a vowel, and you may think the article which must precede it is "an" as in "an airport"; the "u" is pronounced like "you," which starts with a consonant, so the article to be used is "a" instead of "an." In this case you should write:
   - The chairperson of cardiology came from a university hospital.

3. A 22-years-old man presenting ...
   Many times the first sentence of the first slide of a presentation contains the first error. For those lecturers at an intermediate level, this simple mistake is so evident that they barely believe it is one of the most frequent mistakes ever made. It is obvious that the adjective *22-year-old* cannot be written in the plural and it should be written:
   - A 22-year-old man presenting ...

4. There was not biopsy of the graft.
   This is a frequent and relatively subtle mistake made by upper-intermediate speakers. If you still prefer the use of the negative form you should say:
   - There was not any biopsy of the graft.
   But the affirmative form is:
   - There was no biopsy of the graft.

5. It allows to distinguish between ...
   You should use one of the following phrases:
   - It allows us to distinguish between ...
   Or
   - It allows the distinction between ...

6. Please would you tell me where is the cath lab?
   Embedded questions are always troublesome. Whenever a question is embedded in another interrogative sentence its word order changes. This happens when, trying to be polite, we incorrectly change *What time is it?* to *Would you please tell me what time is it?* instead of to *Would you please tell me what time it is?*
   The direct question *Where is the cath lab?* must be transformed to its embedded form as follows:
   - Please would you tell me where the cath lab is?

7. Most of the times cardiac murmurs ...
   You can say *many times* but not *most of the times*. *Most of the time* is correct and you can use *commonly* or *frequently* as equivalent terms.
   Say instead:
   - Most of the time cardiac murmurs ...

8. I look forward to hear from you ...
   This is a very frequent mistake at the end of formal letters such as those sent to editors. The mistake is based upon a grammatical error. *To* may be either a part of the infinitive or a preposition. In this case *to* is not a part of the infinitive of the verb to *hear* but a part of the prepositional verb *look forward to*; it is indeed a preposition.
   There may be irreparable consequences of making this mistake. If you are trying to have an article published in a prestigious journal, then you cannot make formal mistakes, which can preclude the reading of your otherwise-interesting article.
   So instead of *look forward to hear from you*, you should write:
   - I look forward to hearing from you.

9. *Best Regards*
   Although it is used in both academic and informal correspondence *best regards* is a mixture of two strong English collocations: *kind regards* and *best wishes*. In our opinion instead of *best regards*, which is colloquially acceptable, you should write:
   - *Kind regards*
   Or simply
   - *Regards.*

10. Are you suffering from paresthesias?
    Many doctors forget that patients are not colleagues (with some exceptions) and use medical terminology that cannot be understood by them. This technical question would be easily understood in the form:
    - Do you have pins and needles?

11. An European expert on cardiac MR chaired the session.
    Although European starts with a vowel and you may think the article
    which must precede it is "an" as in "an airport," the correct sentence,
    in this case, would be:
    • A European expert on cardiac MR chaired the session.

12. The meeting began a hour ago.
    Although hour starts with a consonant and you may think the article
    that must precede it is "a" as in "a cradle," the correct sentence, in this
    case, would be:
    • The meeting began an hour ago.
    • Words starting with a silent "h" are preceded by "an," as if they
      started with a vowel.

13. The cardiac surgeon who asked for the CMR was operating the stenotic
    aortic valve reported as such by the radiologist.
    This sentence is not correct since the verb "to operate" when is used
    from a surgical point of view (with regard to both patients and parts of
    the anatomy) is always followed by the preposition "on." The correct
    sentence would have been:
    • The cardiac surgeon who asked for the CMR was operating on the
      stenotic aortic valve reported as such by the radiologist.

14. The hospital personal are very kind.
    When we talk about a group of people working at an institution, the
    correct word is "personnel," not "personal":
    • The hospital personnel are very kind.

15. Page to the cardiologist.
    The verb "to page," which could be related to the substantive "page" (a
    boy who is employed to run errands), is not a prepositional verb and
    does not need the preposition "to" after it. When you want the cardiol-
    ogist paged you must say:
    • Page the cardiologist.

16. He works in the neurorradiology division.
    This is a common mistake made by Spanish and Latin American doc-
    tors. In English, neuroradiology is written with one "r":
    • He works in the neuroradiology division.

17. Coronary angiogram revealed reestenosis of the stent.
    The same as stated in the previous numeral, this is a usual mistake
    among Spanish speaking cardiologists. In English, restenosis is written
    with one "e":
    • Coronary angiogram revealed restenosis of the stent.

18. The table shows therapeutic targets and the drugs undergoing assess-
    ment in clinical trials as antirestenotic agents.
    Hyphens should be used to link the words in compound adjectives.

Most of the drugs used in medicine are described by its effects as a compound adjective. So the correct way to write the sentence is:

- The table shows therapeutic targets and the drugs undergoing assessment in clinical trials as anti-restenotic agents.
- Anti-inflammatory, anti-proliferative, anti-arrhythmic, anti-anginal drugs.

19. Young Paula is a very-talented student.
    Linking an adverb like "very" to an adjective with a hyphen is an uncommon error. The correct way to write the phrase is:
    - Young Paula is a very talented student.

20. It was a wonderfully-decorated room.
    When an adverb ends in "ly" (and lots do) some writers feel the urge to link it to the adjective with a hyphen. There is no need because the adverb "wonderfully" modifies the adjective "decorated." The correct form is:
    - It was a wonderfully decorated room.

21. A MR magnet was purchased by the hospital.
    Although *a magnetic resonance magnet ...* is correct, when you use the acronym, do not forget that "m" is read as if it sounded like "em," which begins with a vowel, so the article to be used is "an" instead of "a." In this case you should write:
    - An MR magnet was purchased by the hospital.

Common Spelling Mistakes

Create your own list of potentially misspelled words and do not hesitate to write down your own mnemonic if it helps you.

The following is a list of commonly misspelled words (with the most common misspelling given in parentheses):

- Parallel (misspelled: parallell)
  For this frequently misspelled word, I use this quite absurd (as most mnemonics are) mnemonic to recall the spelling: "Two legs (ll) run faster, and get forward, than one (l)."

- Appearance (misspelled: apearance)
  We have been seen this mistake more than once in cardiological drafts. The only thing you have to check to avoid it is that the verb "appear" is embedded in the word "appearance."

- Sagittal (misspelled: saggital)
  In a word with double consonants and single consonants, avoid doubling the single consonant and vice versa. Sagittal is one of the most commonly misspelled words in slides that show images (MR, CT, and echo).

- Arrhythmia (misspelled: arrythmia)
  Double-check the spelling of arrhythmia and be sure that the word "rhythm," from which it is derived, is embedded in it.

- Severe (misspelled: sever)
  It is frequent in English to find final letters that are not pronounced, leading to the common mistake of omitting them when writing.

Review the following further pairs of words (with the misspelling given in parentheses) and, more importantly, as we said above, create your own list of "troublesome" words.

- Professor (misspelled: proffesor)
- Professional (misspelled: proffesional)
- Occasion (misspelled: ocassion)
- Dissection (misspelled: disection)
- Resection (misspelled: ressection)
- Gray-white matter (misspelled: gray-white mater)
- Subtraction (misspelled: substraction)
- Acquisition (misspelled: adquisition).

Common Pronunciation Mistakes

For simplicity, we have taken the liberty of using an approximate representation of the pronunciation instead of using the phonetic signs. We apologize to our linguist colleagues who may have preferred a more orthodox transcription.

Pronunciation is one of the most dreaded nightmares of English. Although there are pronunciation rules, there are so many exceptions that you must know the pronunciation of most words by ear. Therefore, first, read aloud as much as you can, because it is the only way you will notice the unknown words with regard to pronunciation, and second, when you attend a course, besides concentrating on the presentation itself, focus on the way native English-speaking cardiologists pronounce the words you do not know.

With regard to pronunciation, we recommend that you should:

- Not to be afraid of sounding different or funny. English sounds are different and funny. Sometimes a non-native-speaking cardiologist may know how to pronounce a word correctly but is a bit ashamed of doing so, particularly in the presence of colleagues of the same nationality. Do not be ashamed of pronouncing correctly independently of the nationality of your interlocutor.

- Enjoy the effort of using a different set of muscles in the mouth. In the beginning, the "English muscles" may become stiff and even hurt, but persevere; this is only a sign of hard work.
- Do not worry about having a broad or even embarrassing accent in the beginning; it does not matter as long as you are understood. The idea is to communicate, to say what you think or feel, and not to give a performance in speech therapy.
- Try to pronounce English words properly. As time goes by and you begin to feel relatively confident about your English, we encourage you to progressively and thoroughly study English phonetics. Bear in mind that if you keep your pronunciation as it was at the beginning, then you will sound like American or British people do when speaking your language with their unmistakable accent.
- Rehearse standard collocations in both conversational and cardiological scenarios. Saying straightforward things such as "Do you know what I mean?" or "Would you do me a favor?" and "Who's on call today? Please would you window (and level) this image?" will provide you with extremely useful fluency tools.

Having your own *subtle* national accent in English is not a serious problem as long as the presentation conveys the correct message. However, as far as pronunciation is concerned, there are several tricky words that cannot be properly named false friends and need some extra attention.

In English, some words are spelled differently but sound very much the same. Consider the following, for example:

- *Ileum*: the distal portion of the small intestine, extending from the jejunum to the cecum.
- *Ilium*: the uppermost and widest of the three sections of the hip bone.

Imagine for a moment how surreal it would be for our surgeons to mix up the bowel with the hip bone. Well, we suppose you could say it could be worse – at least both anatomical structures are roughly in the same area!

Again, consider the following:

The English word *tear* means two different things according to how we pronounce it:

- If *tear* (tier) is pronounced, we mean the watery secretion of the lachrymal glands, which serves to moisten the conjunctiva.
- If *tear* (tear) is pronounced, we are referring to the action of wounding or injuring, especially by ripping apart as in "there is a longitudinal *tear* in the posterior leaflet of the tricuspid valve."

Among the cardiological words most commonly mispronounced are two that deserve a close analysis since cardiologists use (or misuse) them almost every single day of their professional lives. These two words are "vascular" and "image."

Many physicians worldwide say they are a specialist in [vas-cu-lar] surgery, "I am a vascular surgeon," instead of [vas-kiu-lar] surgeon. A similar difficulty occurs with intrinsically cardiovascular words such as *cardiovascular, intravascular* ... Please, from now on, avoid this unbelievably frequent mistake.

Image and *images* are two of the most commonly mispronounced medical words. Can you imagine how many times you will see images in your medical life? Please do not say [im-éich] or [im-eiches] but [ím-ich] and [ím-iches]. If you are among the vast group of physicians who used to say [im-éich] for every single slide of every presentation, then do not tell anybody and "keep on" saying [ím-ich] "as you always did." Do not worry! There are probably no records of your presentations, and if they do exist, they are not readily available.

The reason for underlining these two common mistakes is to emphasize that you have to avoid mispronunciation mistakes, beginning with the most usual words in your daily practice. If you are not a chest radiologist and do not know how to pronounce, for example, "lymphangioleiomyomatosis," then don't worry about this word until you have mastered the pronunciation of your day-to-day cardiological terms.

Our piece of advice is, create a top-100 list with your day-to-day most difficult words in terms of spelling. Once you are familiar with them, enlarge your list by keeping on reading out loud as many articles as you can. If you happen to be an interventional cardiologist, brochures and instructions-for-use sheets can keep you posted with virtually no effort and will help you to fill in those useless time-outs between patients.

We have created a list made up of some mispronounced medical words. Since this list is arbitrary and could vary depending on your native tongue, we encourage you to create your own list.

- Parenchyma
  Parenchyma is, in principle, an easy word to pronounce. We include it in this list because we have noticed that some lecturers, particularly Italians, tend to say [pa-ren-kái-ma].

- The letter "h"
  "Non-pronunciation": Italian and French speakers tend to skip this letter, so that when they pronounce the word "enhancement" they say [en-áns-ment] instead of [en-háns-ment]. It is true that "h" can be silent but *not* always.
  "Over-pronunciation": Spanish doctors tend to over-pronounce the letter "h."

- Data
  Although some American doctors say [data], the correct pronunciation of this word is [déi-ta].

- Disease/decease
  The pronunciation of *disease* can be funny, since depending on how you pronounce the "s," you can be saying "decease" which is what terminal diseases end in. The correct pronunciation of *disease* is [di-ssíss] with a liquid "s"; if you say [di-sís] with a plain "s," as many Spanish and Latin American speakers do, every time you talk about, let us say, Alzheimer's disease, you are talking about Alzheimer's decease or Alzheimer's death.

- Chamber
  The pronunciation of *chamber* is somewhat tricky, since French speakers tend "Gallicize" it by saying [cham-bre], whereas some Spanish speakers say simply [cham-ber] instead of [cheim-ber].

- French words as "technique"
  In English you have to say [tek-ník], "in the French way," although you say technical [ték-ni-cal].

- Director
  Although you can say both [di-rect] and [dai-rect] only [dai-rec-tor] is correct; you cannot say [di-rec-tor].

It is beyond the scope of this manual to go over all potentially tricky words in terms of pronunciation, but we offer below a short list of more such words, and would again encourage you to create your own "personal" list.

- Mitral (MÁI-tral)
- Medulla (Me-dú-la)
- Anesthetist (a-nés-te-tist)
- Gynecology (gai-ne-có-lo-gy)
- Edema (i-dima)
- Case report (kéis ri-port, NOT kéis ré-port)
- Multidetector (multi-, NOT mul-tai)
- Oblique (o-blik, NOT o-bláik)
- Femoral (fí-mo-ral)
- Jugular (iu-gu-lar)
- Aortic (ei-ór-tik)

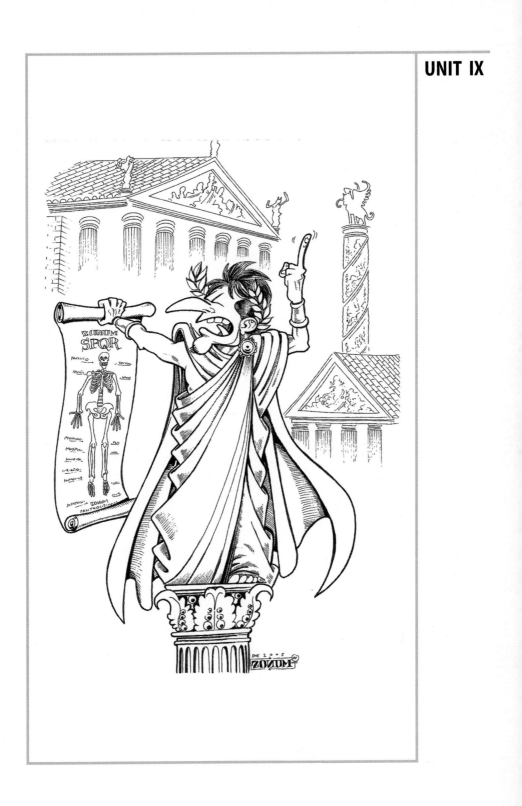

Unit IX Latin and Greek Terminology

Introduction

Latin and Greek terminology is another obstacle to be overcome on the way to becoming fluent in medical English. Romance-language speakers (Spanish, French, Italian, etc.) are undoubtedly at an advantage, although this advantage can become a great drawback in terms of pronunciation and, particularly, in the use of the plural forms of Latin and Greek.

Since most Latin words used in medical English keep the Latin plural ending – e.g., metastasis, *pl.* metastases; viscus, *pl.* viscera – it is essential to understand the basis of plural rules in Latin.

All Latin nouns and adjectives have different endings for each gender (masculine, feminine, or neuter), number (singular or plural), and case – the case is a special ending that reveals the function of the word in a particular sentence. Latin adjectives must correlate with the nouns they modify in case, number, and gender. Although we can barely remember it from our days in high school, there are five different patterns of endings, each one of them is called declension.

The nominative case indicates the subject of a sentence. The genitive case denotes possession or attachment. Dropping the genitive singular ending gives the base to which the nominative plural ending is added to build the medical English plural form.

For example:

- *Corpus* (nominative singular), *corporis* (genitive singular), *corpora* (nominative plural). This is a third-declension neuter noun that means "body." The corresponding forms for the accompanying adjective *callosus* are *callosum*, and *callosa*, respectively. Thus, *corpus callosum* (nominative, singular, neuter), *corpora callosa* (nominative, plural, neuter).

Another example:

- *Coxa vara* (feminine singular), *coxae varae* (feminine plural), but *genu varum* (neuter, singular), *genua vara* (neuter, plural).

Table IX.1. The endings of Latin substantives listed by case and declension

Case	Declension							
	1st	**2nd**		**3rd**		**4th**		**5th**
	Feminine	Masculine	Neuter	Masculine/ feminine	Neuter	Masculine	Neuter	Feminine
Nominative singular	-a	-us	-um			-us	-u	-es
Genitive singular	-ae	-i	-i	-is	-is	-us	-us	-ei
Nominative plural	-ae	-i	-a	-es	-a	-us	-ua	-es

This unit provides an extensive Latin glossary, which includes the singular and plural nominative, and the genitive singular forms of each word, as well as the declension and gender of each word. In some terms, additional items have been added, such as English plural endings when widely accepted (e.g., *fetus*, Latin plural *feti*, English plural *fetuses*), and Greek-origin endings kept in some Latin words (e.g., *thorax*, pl. *thoraces*, gen. *thoracos/thoracis*: chest).

The endings of Latin substantives listed by case and declension are shown in Table IX.1.

Examples:

- 1st declension:
  - Feminine words: *patella* (nom. sing.), *patellae* (gen.), *patellae* (nom. pl). English *patella*

- 2nd declension:
  - Masculine words: *humerus* (nom. sing.), *humeri* (gen.), *humeri* (nom. pl.). English *humerus*
  - Neuter words: *interstitium* (nom. sing.), *interstitii* (gen.), *interstitia* (nom. pl.). English *interstice*

- 3rd declension:
  - Masculine or feminine words: *Pars* (nom. sing.), *partis* (gen.), *partes* (nom. pl.). English *part*
  - Neuter words: *os* (nom. sing.), *oris* (gen.), *ora* (nom. pl.). English *mouth*

- 4th declension:
  - Masculine words: *processus* (nom. sing.), *processus* (gen.), *processus* (nom. pl). English *process*
  - Neuter words: *cornu* (nom. sing.), *cornus* (gen.), *cornua* (nom. pl.). English *horn*

- 5th declension:
  - Feminine words: *facies* (nom. sing.), *faciei* (gen.), *facies* (nom. pl.). English *face*

The endings of the adjectives change according to one of these two patterns:

1. Singular: masc. *-us*, fem. *-a*, neut. *-um*. Plural: masc. *-i*, fem. *-ae*, neut. *-a*
2. Singular: masc. *-is*, fem. *-is*, neut. *-e*. Plural: masc. *-es*, fem. *-es*, neut. *-a*

Plural Rules

It is far from our intention to replace medical dictionaries and Latin or Greek textbooks. Conversely, this unit is aimed at giving some tips related to Latin and Greek terminology, which can provide a consistent approach to this challenging topic.

Our first piece of advice on this subject is that whenever you write a Latin or Greek word, first, check its spelling, and, second, if the word you want to write is a plural one, never make it up. Although guessing the plural form could be acceptable as an exercise in itself, double-check the word by looking it up in a medical dictionary.

The following plural rules are useful to give at least us self-confidence in the use of usual Latin or Greek terms such as *metastasis–metastases, pelvis–pelves, bronchus–bronchi*, etc.

Some overseas doctors do think that *metastasis* and *metastases* are equivalent terms, and they are absolutely wrong; the difference between a unique liver metastasis and multiple liver metastases is so obvious that no additional comment is needed.

There are many Latin and Greek words whose singular forms are almost never used, as well as Latin and Greek terms whose plural forms are seldom said or written. Let us think, for example, about the singular form of *viscera* (*viscus*). Very few physicians are aware that the liver is a *viscus*, whereas the liver and spleen are *viscera*. From a colloquial standpoint, this discussion might be considered futile, but those who write papers do know that Latin/Greek terminology is always a nightmare and needs thorough revision, and that terms seldom used on a day-to-day basis have to be properly written in a scientific article. Again, let us consider the plural form of *pelvis* (*pelves*). To talk about several pelves is so rare that many doctors have never wondered what the plural form of pelvis is.

Although there are some exceptions, the following general rules can be helpful with plural terms:

- Words ending in *-us* change to *-i* (2nd declension masculine words):
  - *Bronchus* → *bronchi*

- Words ending in -*um* change to -*a* (2nd declension neuter words):
  - *Acetabulum* → *acetabula*
- Words ending in -*a* change to -*ae* (1st declension feminine words):
  - *Vena* → *venae*
- Words ending in -*ma* change to -*mata* or -*mas* (3rd declension neuter words of Greek origin):
  - *Sarcoma* → *sarcomata/sarcomas*
- Words ending in -*is* change to -*es* (3rd declension masculine or feminine words):
  - *Metastasis* → *metastases*
- Words ending in -*itis* change to -*itides* (3rd declension masculine or feminine words):
  - *Arthritis* → *arthritides*
- Words ending in -*x* change to -*ces* (3rd declension masculine or feminine words):
  - *Pneumothorax* → *pneumothoraces*
- Words ending in -*cyx* change to -*cyges* (3rd declension masculine or feminine words):
  - *Coccyx* → *coccyges*
- Words ending in -*ion* change to -*ia* (2nd declension neuter words, most of Greek origin):
  - *Criterion* → *criteria*

List of Latin and Greek Terms and Their Plurals

Abbreviations:
adj.   adjective
Engl.   English
fem.   feminine
gen.   genitive
Gr.   Greek
Lat.   Latin
lit.   literally
m.   muscle
masc.   masculine
neut.   neuter
pl.   plural
sing.   singular

A

- **Abdomen**, pl. **abdomina**, gen. **abdominis**. Abdomen. 3rd declension neut.
- **Abducens**, pl. **abducentes**, gen. **abducentis** (from the verb *abduco*, to detach, to lead away)
- **Abductor**, pl. **abductores**, gen. **abductoris** (from the verb *abduco*, to detach, to lead away). 3rd declension masc.
- **Acetabulum**, pl. **acetabula**, gen. **acetabuli**. Cotyle. 2nd declension neut.
- **Acinus**, pl. **acini**, gen. **acini**. Acinus. 2nd declension masc.
- **Adductor**, pl. **adductores**, gen. **adductoris**. Adductor. 3rd declension masc.
- **Aditus,** pl. **aditus**, gen. **aditus**. Entrance to a cavity. 4th declension masc.
  – *Aditus ad antrum, aditus glottidis inferior,* etc.
- **Agger**, pl. **aggeres**, gen. **aggeris**. Agger (prominence). 3rd declension masc.
  – *Agger valvae venae, agger nasi, agger perpendicularis,* etc.
- **Ala**, pl. **alae**, gen. **alae**. Wing. 1st declension fem.
- **Alveolus**, pl. **alveoli**, gen. **alveoli**. Alveolus (lit. *basin*). 2nd declension masc.
- **Alveus**, pl. **alvei**, gen. **alvei**. Cavity, hollow. 2nd declension masc.
- **Amoeba**, pl. **amoebae**, gen. **amoebae**. Ameba. 1st declension fem.
- **Ampulla**, pl. **ampullae**, gen. **ampullae**. Ampoule, blister. 1st declension fem.
- **Anastomosis**, pl. **anastomoses**, gen. **anastomosis**. Anastomosis. 3rd declension.
- **Angulus**, pl. **anguli**, gen. **anguli**. Angle, apex, corner. 2nd declension neut.
- **Annulus**, pl. **annuli**, gen. **annuli**. Ring. 2nd declension masc.
- **Ansa**, pl. **ansae**, gen. **ansae**. Loop, hook, handle. 1st declension fem.
- **Anterior**, pl. **anteriores**, gen. **anterioris**. Foremost, that is before, former. 3rd declension masc.
- **Antrum**, pl. **antra**, gen. **antri**. Antrum, hollow, cave. 2nd declension neut.
- **Anus**, pl. **ani**, gen. **ani**. Anus (lit. *ring*). 2nd declension masc.
- **Aorta**, pl. **Aortae**, gen. **aortae**. Aorta. 1st declension fem.
- **Apex**, pl. **apices**, gen. **apices**. Apex (top, summit, cap). 3rd declension masc.
- **Aphtha**, pl. **aphthae**, gen. **aphthae**. Aphtha (small ulcer). 1st declension fem.
- **Aponeurosis**, pl. **aponeuroses**, gen. **aponeurosis**. Aponeurosis. 3rd. declension
- **Apophysis**, pl. **apophyses**, gen. **apophysos/apophysis**. Apophysis. 3rd declension fem.
- **Apparatus**, pl. **apparatus**, gen. **apparatus**. Apparatus, system. 4th declension masc.
- **Appendix**, pl. **appendices**, gen. **appendicis**. Appendage. 3rd declension fem.

- **Area**, pl. **areae**, gen. **areae**. Area. 1st declension fem.
- **Areola**, pl. **areolae**, gen. **areolae**. Areola (lit. *little area*). 1st declension fem.
- **Arrector**, pl. **arrectores**, gen. **arrectoris**. Erector, tilt upwards. 3rd declension masc.
- **Arteria**, pl. **arteriae**, gen. **arteriae**. Artery. 1st declension fem.
- **Arteriola**, pl. **arteriolae**, gen. **arteriolae**. Arteriola (small artery). 1st declension fem.
- **Arthritis**, pl. **arthritides**, gen. **arthritidis**. Arthritis. 3rd declension fem.
- **Articularis**, pl. **articulares**, gen. **articularis**. Articular, affecting the joints. 3rd declension masc. (adj.: masc. *articularis*, fem. *articularis*, neut. *articulare*)
- **Articulatio**, pl. **articulationes**, gen. **articulationis**. Joint. 3rd declension fem.
- **Atlas**, pl. **atlantes**, gen. **atlantis**. First cervical vertebra. 3rd declension masc.
- **Atrium**, pl. **atria**, gen. **atrii**. Atrium. 2nd declension neut.
- **Auricula**, pl. **auriculae**, gen. **auriculae**. Auricula (ear flap). 1st declension fem.
- **Auricularis m.**, pl. **auriculares**, gen. **auricularis**. Pertaining to the ear. 3rd declension masc.
- **Auris**, pl. **aures**, gen. **auris**. Ear. 3rd declension fem.
- **Axilla**, pl. **axillae**, gen. **axillae**. Armpit. 1st declension fem.
- **Axis**, pl. **axes**, gen. **axis**. Second cervical vertebra, axis. 3rd declension masc.

B
- **Bacillus**, pl. **bacilli**, gen. **bacilli**. Stick-shape bacterium (lit. *small stick*). 2nd declension masc.
- **Bacterium**, pl. **bacteria**, gen. **bacterii**. Bacterium. 2nd declension neut.
- **Basis**, pl. **bases**, gen. **basis**. Basis, base. 3rd declension fem.
- **Biceps m.**, pl. **bicipites**, gen. **bicipitis**. A muscle with two heads. 3rd declension masc.
  - Biceps + genitive. Biceps *brachii* (*brachium*. Arm)
- **Borborygmus**, pl. **borborygmi**, gen. **borborygmi**. Borborygmus (gastrointestinal sound). 2nd declension masc.
- **Brachium**, pl. **brachia**, gen. **brachii**. Arm. 2nd declension neut.
- **Brevis**, pl. **breves**, gen. **brevis**. Short, little, small. 3rd declension masc. (adj.: masc. *brevis*, fem. *brevis*, neut. *breve*)
- **Bronchium**, pl. **bronchia**, gen. **bronchii**. Bronchus. 2nd declension neut.
- **Buccinator m.**, pl. **buccinatores**, gen. **buccinatoris**. Buccinator m. (trumpeter's muscle). 3rd declension masc.
- **Bulla**, pl. **bullae**, gen. **bullae**. Bulla. 1st declension fem.
- **Bursa**, pl. **bursae**, gen. **bursae**. Bursa (bag, pouch). 1st declension fem.

C

- **Caecum**, pl. **caeca**, gen. **caeci**. Blind. 2nd declension neut. (adj.: masc. *caecus*, fem. *caeca*, neut. *caecum*)
- **Calcaneus**, pl. **calcanei**, gen. **calcanei**. Calcaneus (from *calx*, heel). 2nd declension masc.
- **Calculus**, pl. **calculi**, gen. **calculi**. Stone (lit. pebble). 2nd declension masc.
- **Calix**, pl. **calices**, gen. **calicis**. Calix (lit. *cup, goblet*). 3rd declension masc.
- **Calx**, pl. **calces**, gen. **calcis**. Heel. 3rd declension masc.
- **Canalis**, pl. **canales**, gen. **canalis**. Channel, conduit. 3rd declension masc.
- **Cancellus**, pl. **cancelli**, gen. **cancelli**. Reticulum, lattice, grid. 2nd declension masc.
- **Cancer**, pl. **cancera**, gen. **canceri**. Cancer. 3rd declension neut.
- **Capillus**, pl. **capilli**, gen. **capilli**. Hair. 2nd declension masc.
- **Capitatus**, pl. **capitati**, gen. **capitati**. Capitate, having or forming a head. 2nd declension masc. (adj.: masc. *capitatus*, fem. *capitata*, neut. *capitatum*)
- **Capitulum**, pl. **capitula**, gen. **capituli**. Head of a structure, condyle. 2nd declension neut.
- **Caput**, pl. **capita**, gen. **capitis**. Head. 3rd declension neut.
- **Carcinoma**, pl. Lat. **carcinomata**, pl. Engl. **carcinomas**, gen. **carcinomatis**. Carcinoma (epithelial cancer). 3rd declension neut.
- **Carina**, pl. **carinae**, gen. **carinae**. Carina (lit. *keel, bottom of ship*). 1st declension fem.
- **Cartilago**, pl. **cartilagines**, gen. **cartilaginis**. Cartilage. 3rd declension neut.
- **Cauda**, pl. **caudae**, gen. **caudae**. Tail. 1st declension fem.
  - *Cauda equina* (adj.: masc. *equinus*, fem. *equina*, neut. *equinum*. Concerning horses)
- **Caverna**, pl. **cavernae**, gen. **cavernae**. Cavern. 1st declension fem.
- **Cavitas**, pl. **cavitates**, gen. **cavitatis**. Cavity. 3rd declension fem.
- **Cavum**, pl. **cava**, gen. **cavi**. Cavum (hole, pit, depression). 2nd declension neut.
- **Cella**, pl. **cellae**, gen. **cellae**. Cell (lit. *cellar, wine storeroom*). 1st declension fem.
- **Centrum**, pl. **centra**, gen. **centri**. Center. 2nd declension neut.
- **Cerebellum**, pl. **cerebella**, gen. **cerebelli**. Cerebellum. 2nd declension neut.
- **Cerebrum**, pl. **cerebra**, gen. **cerebri**. Brain. 2nd declension neut.
- **Cervix**, pl. **cervices**, gen. **cervicis**. Neck. 3rd declension fem.
- **Chiasma**, pl. **chiasmata**, gen. **chiasmatis/chiasmatos**. Chiasm. 3rd declension neut.
- **Choana**, pl. **choanae**, gen. **choanae**. Choana. 1st declension fem.
  - *Choanae narium*. Posterior opening of the nasal fossae (*naris*, gen. *narium*. nose)

- **Chorda**, pl. **chordae**, gen. **chordae**. String. 1st declension fem.
  - *Chorda tympani*. A nerve given off from the facial nerve in the facial canal that crosses over the tympanic membrane (*tympanum*, gen. *tympani*. eardrum)
- **Chorion**, pl. **choria**, gen. **chorii**. Chorion (membrane enclosing the fetus). 2nd declension neut.
- **Cicatrix**, pl. **cicatrices**, gen. **cicatricis**. Scar. 3rd declension fem.
- **Cilium**, pl. **cilia**, gen. **cilii**. Cilium (lit. *upper eyelid*). 2nd declension neut.
- **Cingulum**, pl. **cingula**, gen. **cinguli**. Cingulum (belt-shaped structure, lit. *belt*). 2nd declension neut.
- **Cisterna**, pl. **cisternae**, gen. **cisternae**. Cistern. 1st declension fem.
- **Claustrum**, pl. **claustra**, gen. **claustri**. Claustrum. 2nd declension neut.
- **Clitoris**, pl. **clitorides**, gen. **clitoridis**. Clitoris. 3rd declension
- **Clivus**, pl. **clivi**, gen. **clivi**. Clivus (part of the skull, lit. *slope*). 2nd declension masc.
- **Clostridium**, pl. **clostridia**, gen. **clostridii**. *Clostridium* (genus of bacteria). 2nd declension neut.
- **Coccus**, pl. **cocci**, gen. **cocci**. Coccus (rounded bacterium, lit. *a scarlet dye*). 2nd declension masc.
- **Coccyx**, pl. **coccyges**, gen. **coccygis**. Coccyx. 3rd declension masc.
- **Cochlea**, pl. **cochleae**, gen. **cochleae**. Cochlea (lit. *snail shell*). 1st declension fem.
- **Collum**, pl. **colla**, gen. **colli**. Neck. 2nd declension neut.
- **Comedo**, pl. **comedones**, gen. **comedonis**. Comedo (a dilated hair follicle filled with keratin). 3rd declension masc.
- **Comunis**, pl. **comunes**, gen. **comunis**. Common. 3rd declension masc. (adj.: masc./fem. *comunis*, neut. *comune*)
- **Concha**, pl. **conchae**, gen. **conchae**. Concha (shell-shaped structure). 1st declension fem.
- **Condyloma**, pl. **condylomata**, gen. **condylomatis**. Condyloma. 3rd declension neut.
  - *Condyloma acuminatum*
- **Conjunctiva**, pl. **conjunctivae**, gen. **conjunctivae**. Conjunctiva. 1st declension fem.
- **Constrictor**, pl. **constrictores**, gen. **constrictoris**. Sphincter. 3rd declension masc.
- **Conus**, pl. **coni**, gen. **coni**. Cone. 2nd declension masc.
  - *Conus medullaris* (from *medulla*, pl. *medullae*, the tapering end of the spinal cord).
- **Cor**, pl. **corda**, gen. **cordis**. Heart. 3rd declension neut.
- **Corium**, pl. **coria**, gen. **corii**. Dermis (lit. *skin*). 2nd declension neut.
- **Cornu**, pl. **Cornua**, gen. **cornus**. Horn. 4th declension neut.
- **Corona**, pl. **coronae**, gen. **coronae**. Corona (lit. *crown*). 1st declension fem.
  - *Corona radiata*, pl. *coronae radiatae*, gen. *coronae radiatae*

- **Corpus**, pl. **corpora**, gen. **corporis**. Body. 3rd declension neut.
  - *Corpus callosum, corpus cavernosum* (penis)
- **Corpusculum**, pl. **corpuscula**, gen. **corpusculi**. Corpuscle. 2nd declension neut.
- **Cortex**, pl. **cortices**, gen. **corticis**. Cortex, outer covering. 3rd declension masc.
- **Coxa**, pl. **coxae**, gen. **coxae**. Hip. 1st declension fem.
- **Cranium**, pl. **crania**, gen. **cranii**. Skull. 2nd declension neut.
- **Crisis**, pl. **crises**, gen. **crisos/crisis**. Crisis. 3rd declension fem.
- **Crista**, pl. **cristae**, gen. **cristae**. Crest. 1st declension fem.
  - *Crista galli* (from *gallus*, pl. *galli*, rooster. The midline process of the ethmoid bone arising from the cribriform plate).
- **Crus**, pl. **crura**, gen. **cruris**. Leg, leg-like structure. 3rd declension neut.
  - *Crura diaphragmatis*
- **Crusta**, pl. **crustae**, gen. **crustae**. Crust, hard surface. 1st declension fem.
- **Crypta**, pl. **cryptae**, gen. **cryptae**. Crypt. 1st declension fem.
- **Cubitus**, pl. **cubiti**, gen. **cubiti**. Ulna (lit. *forearm*). 2nd declension masc.
- **Cubitus**, pl. **cubitus**, gen. **cubitus**. State of lying down. 4th declension masc.
  - *De cubito supino/prono*
- **Culmen**, pl. **culmina**, gen. **culminis**. Peak, top (*culmen*. Top of cerebellar lobe). 3rd declension neut.
- **Cuneiforme**, pl. **cuneiformia**, gen. **cuneiformis**. Wedge-shaped structure. 3rd declension neut. (adj.: masc. *cuneiformis*, fem. *cuneiformis*, neut. *cuneiforme*)

D

- **Decussatio**, pl. **decussationes**, gen. **decussationis**. Decussation. 3rd declension fem.
- **Deferens**, pl. **deferentes**, gen. **deferentis**. Spermatic duct (from the verb *defero*, to carry). 3rd declension masc.
- **Dens**, pl. **dentes**, gen. **dentis**. Tooth, pl. Teeth. 3rd declension masc.
- **Dermatitis**, pl. **dermatitides**, gen. **dermatitis**. Dermatitis. 3rd declension.
- **Dermatosis**, pl. **dermatoses**, gen. **dermatosis**. Dermatosis. 3rd declension.
- **Diaphragma**, pl. **diaphragmata**, gen. **diaphragmatis**. Diaphragm. 3rd declension neut.
- **Diaphysis**, pl. **Diaphyses**, gen. **diaphysis**. Shaft. 3rd declension.
- **Diarthrosis**, pl. **diarthroses**, gen. **diarthrosis**. Diarthrosis. 3rd declension.
- **Diastema**, pl. **diastemata**, gen. **diastematis**. Diastema (congenital fissure). 3rd declension.
- **Digastricus m.**, pl. **digastrici**, gen. **digastrici**. Digastric (having two bellies). 2nd declension masc.

- **Digitus**, pl. **digiti**, gen. sing. **digiti**, gen. pl. **digitorum**. Finger. 2nd declension masc.
  - *Extensor digiti minimi, flexor superficialis digitorum*
- **Diverticulum**, pl. **diverticula**, gen. **diverticuli**. Diverticulum. 2nd declension neut.
- **Dorsum**, pl. **dorsa**, gen. **dorsi**. Back. 2nd declension neut.
- **Ductus**, pl. **ductus**, gen. **ductus**. Duct. 4th declension masc.
  - *Ductus arteriosus, ductus deferens*
- **Duodenum**, pl. **duodena**, gen. **duodeni**. Duodenum (lit. *twelve*. The duodenum measures 12 times a finger). 2nd declension neut.

E

- **Ecchymosis**, pl. **ecchymoses**, gen. **ecchymosis**. Ecchymosis. 3rd declension.
- **Effluvium**, pl. **effluvia**, gen. **effluvii**. Effluvium (fall). 2nd declension neut.
- **Encephalitis**, pl. **encephalitides**, gen. **encephalitidis**. Encephalitis. 3rd declension fem.
- **Endocardium**, pl. **endocardia**, gen. **endocardii**. Endocardium. 2nd declension neut.
- **Endometrium**, pl. **endometria**, gen. **endometrii**. Endometrium. 2nd declension neut.
- **Endothelium**, pl. **endothelia**, gen. **endothelii**. Endothelium. 2nd declension neut.
- **Epicondylus**, pl. **epicondyli**, gen. **epicondyli**. Epicondylus. 2nd declension masc.
- **Epidermis**, pl. **epidermides**, gen. **epidermidis**. Epidermis. 3rd declension.
- **Epididymis**, pl. **epididymes**, gen. **epididymis**. Epididymis. 3rd declension.
- **Epiphysis**, pl. **epiphyses**, gen. **epiphysis**. Epiphysis. 3rd declension.
- **Epithelium**, pl. **epithelia**, gen. **epithelii**. Epithelium. 2nd declension neut.
- **Esophagus**, pl. **esophagi**, gen. **esophagi**. Esophagus. 2nd declension masc.
- **Exostosis**, pl. **exostoses**, gen. **exostosis**. Exostosis. 3rd declension.
- **Extensor**, pl. **extensores**, gen. **extensoris**. A muscle contraction of which stretches out a structure. 3rd declension masc.
  - *Extensor carpi ulnaris m., extensor digitorum communis m., extensor hallucis longus/brevis m.*, etc.
- **Externus**, pl. **externi**, gen. **externi**. External, outward. 2nd declension masc. (adj.: masc. *externus*, fem. *externa*, gen. *externum*)

F

- **Facies**, pl. **facies**, gen. **faciei**. Face. 5th declension fem.
- **Falx**, pl. **falces**, gen. **falcis**. Sickle-shaped structure. 3rd declension fem.
  - *Falx cerebrii*
- **Fascia**, pl. **fasciae**, gen. **fasciae**. Fascia. 1st declension fem.
- **Fasciculus**, pl. **fasciculi**, gen. **fasciculi**. Fasciculus. 2nd declension masc.
- **Femur**, pl. **femora**, gen. **femoris**. Femur. 3rd declension neut.
- **Fenestra**, pl. **fenestrae**, gen. **fenestrae**. Window, hole. 1st declension fem.
- **Fetus**, pl. **feti/fetus**, gen. **feti/fetus**. Fetus. 2nd declension masc./4th declension masc.
- **Fibra**, pl. **fibrae**, gen. **fibrae**. Fiber. 1st declension fem.
- **Fibula**, pl. **fibulae**, gen. **fibulae**. Fibula. 1st declension fem.
- **Filamentum**, pl. **filamenta**, gen. **filamentii**. Filament. 2nd declension neut.
- **Filaria**, pl. **filariae**, gen. **filariae**. Filaria. 1st declension fem.
- **Filum**, pl. **fila**, gen. **fili**. Filamentous structure. 2nd declension neut.
  - *Filum terminale*
- **Fimbria**, pl. **fimbriae**, gen. **fimbriae**. Fimbria (lit. *fringe*). 1st declension fem.
- **Fistula**, pl. **fistulae**, gen. **fistulae**. Fistula (lit. *pipe, tube*). 1st declension fem.
- **Flagellum**, pl. **flagella**, gen. **flagelli**. Flagellum (whip-like locomotory organelle). 2nd declension neut.
- **Flexor**, pl. **flexores**, gen. **flexoris**. A muscle whose action flexes a joint. 3rd declension masc.
  - *Flexor carpi radialis/ulnaris mm., flexor pollicis longus/brevis mm.,* etc.
- **Flexura**, pl. **flexurae**, gen. **flexurae**. Flexure, curve, bow. 1st declension fem.
- **Folium**, pl. **folia**, gen. **folii**. Leaf-shaped structure (lit. *leaf*). 2nd declension neut.
- **Folliculus**, pl. **folliculi**, gen. **folliculi**. Follicle. 2nd declension masc.
- **Foramen**, pl. **foramina**, gen. **foraminis**. Foramen, hole. 3rd declension neut.
  - *Foramen rotundum, foramen ovale*
  - *Foramina cribrosa*, pl. (multiple pores in lamina cribrosa)
- **Formula**, pl. **formulae**, gen. **formulae**. Formula. 1st declension fem.
- **Fornix**, pl. **fornices**, gen. **fornicis**. Fornix (arch-shaped structure). 3rd declension masc.
- **Fossa**, pl. **fossae**, gen. **fossae**. Fossa, depression. 1st declension fem.
- **Fovea**, pl. **foveae**, gen. **foveae**. Fovea, depression, pit. 1st declension fem.
- **Frenulum**, pl. **frenula**, gen. **frenuli**. Bridle-like structure. 2nd declension neut.
- **Fungus**, pl. **fungi**, gen. **fungi**. Fungus (lit. *mushroom*). 2nd declension masc.
- **Funiculus**, pl. **funiculi**, gen. **funiculi**. Cord, string. 2nd declension masc.

- **Furfur**, pl. **furfures**, gen. **furfuris**. Dandruff. 3rd declension masc.
- **Furunculus**, pl. **furunculi**, gen. **furunculi**. Furuncle. 2nd declension masc.

G

- **Galea**, pl. **galeae**, gen. **galeae**. Cover, a structure shaped like a helmet (lit. *helmet*). 1st declension fem.
  - *Galea aponeurotica*, pl. *galeae aponeuroticae* (epicranial aponeurosis)
- **Ganglion**, pl. **ganglia**, gen. **ganglii**. Node. 2nd declension masc.
- **Geniculum**, pl. **genicula**, gen. **geniculi**. Geniculum (knee-shaped structure). 2nd declension neut.
- **Geniohyoideus m.**, pl. **geniohyoidei**, gen. **geniohyoidei**. Glenohyoid muscle. 2nd declension masc.
- **Genu**, pl. **genua**, gen. **genus**. Knee. 4th declension neut.
- **Genus**, pl. **genera**, gen. **generis**. Gender. 3rd declension neut.
- **Gestosis**, pl. **gestoses**, gen. **gestosis**. Gestosis (pregnancy impairment). 3rd declension.
- **Gingiva**, pl. **gingivae**, gen. **gingivae**. Gum. 1st declension fem.
- **Glabella**, pl. **glabellae**, gen. **glabellae**. Small lump/mass. 1st declension fem.
- **Glandula**, pl. **glandulae**, gen. **glandulae**. Gland. 1st declension fem.
- **Glans**, pl. **glandes**, gen. **glandis**. Glans (lit. *acorn*). 3rd declension fem.
  - *Glans penis*
- **Globus**, pl. **globi**, gen. **globi**. Globus, round body. 2nd declension masc.
- **Glomerulus**, pl. **glomeruli**, gen. **glomeruli**. Glomerule. 2nd declension masc.
- **Glomus**, pl. **glomera**, gen. **glomeris**. Glomus (ball-shaped body). 3rd declension.
- **Glottis**, pl. **glottides**, gen. **glottidis**. Glottis. 3rd declension.
- **Gluteus m.**, pl. **glutei**, gen. **glutei**. Buttock. 2nd declension masc.
- **Gracilis m.**, pl. **graciles**, gen. **gracilis**. Graceful. 3rd declension masc. (adj.: masc. *gracilis*, fem. *gracilis*, neut. *gracile*)
- **Granulatio**, pl. **granulationes**, gen. **granulationis**. Granulation. 3rd declension.
- **Gumma**, pl. **gummata**, gen. **gummatis**. Syphiloma. 3rd declension neut.
- **Gutta**, pl. **guttae**, gen. **guttae**. Gout. 1st declension fem.
- **Gyrus**, pl. **gyri**, gen. **gyri**. Convolution. 2nd declension masc.
  Gastrocnemius m., pl. **gastrocnemii**, gen. **gastrocnemii**. Calf muscle. 2nd declension masc.

H

- **Hallux**, pl. **halluces**, gen. **hallucis**. First toe. 3rd declension masc.
- **Hamatus**, pl. **hamati**, gen. **hamati**. Hamate bone. 2nd declension masc. (adj.: masc. *hamatus*, fem. *hamata*, neut. *hamatum*. Hooked)
- **Hamulus**, pl. **hamuli**, gen. **hamuli**. Hamulus (lit. *small hook*). 2nd declension masc.

- **Haustrum**, pl. **haustra**, gen. **haustri**. Pouch from the lumen of the colon. 2nd declension neut.
- **Hiatus**, pl. **hiatus**, gen. **hiatus**. Gap, cleft. 4th declension masc.
- **Hilum**, pl. **hila**, gen. **hili**. Hilum (the part of an organ where the neurovascular bundle enters). 2nd declension neut.
- **Hircus**, pl. **hirci**, gen. **hirci**. Hircus (armpit hair, lit. *goat*). 2nd declension masc.
- **Humerus**, pl. **humeri**, gen. **humeri**. Humerus. 2nd declension masc.
- **Humor**, pl. **humores**, gen. **humoris**. Humor, fluid. 3rd declension masc.
- **Hypha**, pl. **hyphae**, gen. **hyphae**. Hypha, tubular cell (lit. Gr. *web*). 1st declension fem.
- **Hypophysis**, pl. **hypophyses**, gen. **hypophysis**. Pituitary gland (lit. *undergrowth*). 3rd declension.
- **Hypothenar**, pl. **hypothenares**, gen. **hypothenaris**. Hypothenar (from Gr. *thenar*, the palm of the hand). 3rd declension.

I

- **Ilium**, pl. **ilia**, gen. **ilii**. Iliac bone. 2nd declension neut.
- **In situ**. In position (from *situs*, pl. *situs*, gen. *situs*, site). 4th declension masc.
- **Incisura**, pl. **incisurae**, gen. **incisurae**. Incisure (from the verb *incido*, cut into). 1st declension fem.
- **Incus**, pl. **incudes**, gen. **incudis**. Incus (lit. *anvil*). 3rd declension fem.
- **Index**, pl. **indices**, gen. **indicis**. Index (second digit, forefinger), guide. 3rd declension masc.
- **Indusium**, pl. **indusia**, gen. **indusii**. Indusium (membrane, amnion). 2nd declension neut.
- **Inferior**, pl. **inferiores**, gen. **inferioris**. Inferior. 3rd declension masc.
- **Infundibulum**, pl. **infundibula**, gen. **infundibuli**. Infundibulum. 2nd declension neut.
- **Insula**, pl. **insulae**, gen. **insulae**. Insula. 1st declension fem.
- **Intermedius**, pl. **intermedii**, gen. **intermedii**. In the middle of. 2nd declension masc. (adj.: masc. *intermedius*, fem. *intermedia*, neut. *intermedium*)
- **Internus**, pl. **interni**, gen. **interni**. Internal. 2nd declension masc. (adj.: masc. *internus*, fem. *interna*, neut. *internum*)
- **Interosseus**, gen. **interossei**, pl. **interossei**. Interosseous. 2nd declension masc. (adj.: masc. *interosseus*, fem. *interossea*, neut. *interosseum*)
- **Intersectio**, pl. **intersectiones**, gen. **intersectionis**. Intersection. 3rd declension fem.
- **Interstitium**, pl. **interstitia**, gen. **interstitii**. Interstice. 2nd declension neut.
- **Intestinum**, pl. **intestina**, gen. **intestini**. Bowel. 2nd declension neut.
- **Iris**, pl. **irides**, gen. **iridis**. Iris. 3rd declension masc.
- **Ischium**, pl. **ischia**, gen. **ischii**. Ischium. 2nd declension neut.
- **Isthmus**, pl. Lat. **isthmi**, pl. Engl. **isthmuses**, gen. **isthmi**. Constriction, narrow passage. 2nd declension masc.

J

- **Jejunum**, pl. **jejuna**, gen. **jejuni**. Jejunum (from Lat. adj. *jejunus*, fasting, empty). 2nd declension neut.
- **Jugular**, pl. **jugulares**, gen. **jugularis**. Jugular vein (lit. relating to the throat, from Lat. *jugulus*, throat). 3rd declension.
- **Junctura**, pl. **juncturae**, gen. **juncturae**. Joint, junction. 1st declension fem.

L

- **Labium**, pl. **labia**, gen. **labii**. Lip. 2nd declension neut.
- **Labrum**, pl. **labra**, gen. **labri**. Rim, edge, lip. 2nd declension neut.
- **Lacuna**, pl. **lacunae**, gen. **lacunae**. Pond, pit, hollow. 1st declension fem.
- **Lamellipodium**, pl. **lamellipodia**, gen. **lamellipodii**. Lamellipodium. 2nd declension neut.
- **Lamina**, pl. **laminae**, gen. **laminae**. Layer. 1st declension fem.
  - *Lamina papyracea, lamina perpendicularis*
- **Larva**, pl. **larvae**, gen. **larvae**. Larva. 1st declension fem.
- **Larynx**, pl. Lat. **larynges**, pl. Engl. **larynxes**, gen. **laryngis**. Larynx. 3rd declension.
- **Lateralis**, pl. **laterales**, gen. **lateralis**. Lateral. 3rd declension masc. (adj.: masc. *lateralis*, fem. *lateralis*, neut. *laterale*)
- **Latissimus**, pl. **latissimi**, gen. **latissimi**. Very wide, the widest. 2nd declension masc. (adj.: masc. *latissimus*, fem. *latissima*, neut. *latissimum*)
- **Latus**, pl. **latera**, gen. **lateris**. Flank. 3rd declension neut.
- **Latus**, pl. **lati**, gen. **lati**. Wide, broad. 2nd declension masc. (adj.: masc. *latus*, fem. *lata*, neut. *latum*)
- **Lemniscus**, pl. **lemnisci**, gen. **lemnisci**. Lemniscus (lit. *ribbon*). 2nd declension masc.
- **Lentigo**, pl. **lentigines**, gen. **lentiginis**. Lentigo (lit. *lentil-shaped spot*). 3rd declension.
- **Levator**, pl. **levatores**, gen. **levatoris**. Lifter (from Lat. verb *levo*, to lift). 3rd declension masc.
- **Lien**, pl. **lienes**, gen. **lienis**. Spleen. 3rd declension masc.
- **Lienculus**, pl. **lienculi**, gen. **lienculi**. Accessory spleen. 2nd declension masc.
- **Ligamentum**, pl. **ligamenta**, gen. **ligamenti**. Ligament. 2nd declension neut.
- **Limbus**, pl. **limbi**, gen. **limbi**. Border, edge. 2nd declension masc.
- **Limen**, pl. **limina**, gen. **liminis**. Threshold. 3rd declension neut.
- **Linea**, pl. **lineae**, gen. **lineae**. Line. 1st declension fem.
- **Lingua**, pl. **linguae**, gen. **linguae**. Tongue. 1st declension fem.
- **Lingualis**, pl. **linguales**, gen. **lingualis**. Relative to the tongue. 3rd declension masc. (adj.: masc. *lingualis*, fem. *lingualis*, neut. *linguale*)
- **Lingula**, pl. **lingulae**, gen. **lingulae**. Lingula (tongue-shaped). 1st declension fem.
- **Liquor**, pl. **liquores**, gen. **liquoris**. Fluid. 3rd declension masc.

- **Lobulus**, pl. **lobuli**, gen. **lobuli**. Lobule. 2nd declension masc.
- **Lobus**, pl. **lobi**, gen. **lobi**. Lobe. 2nd declension masc.
- **Loculus**, pl. **loculi**, gen. **loculi**. Loculus (small chamber). 2nd declension masc.
- **Locus**, pl. **loci**, gen. **loci**. Locus (place, position, point). 2nd declension masc.
- **Longissimus**, pl. **longissimi**, gen. **longissimi**. Very long, the longest. 2nd declension masc. (adj.: masc. longissimus, fem. longissima, neut. longissimum)
  - *Longissimus dorsi/capitis mm.* (long muscle of the back/head)
- **Longus**, pl. **longi**, gen. **longi**. Long. 2nd declension masc. (adj.: masc. *longus*, fem. *longa*, neut. *longum*)
  - *Longus colli m.* (long muscle of the neck)
- **Lumbar**, pl. **lumbares**, gen. **lumbaris**. Lumbar. 3rd declension.
- **Lumbus**, pl. **lumbi**, gen. **lumbi**. Loin. 2nd declension masc.
- **Lumen**, pl. **lumina**, gen. **luminis**. Lumen. 3rd declension neut.
- **Lunatum**, pl. **lunata**, gen. **lunati**. Lunate bone, crescent-shaped structure. 2nd declension neut. (adj.: masc. *lunatus*, fem. *lunata*, neut. *lunatum*)
  Lunula, pl. lunulae, gen. lunulae. Lunula. 1st declension fem.
- **Lymphonodus**, pl. **lymphonodi**, gen. **lymphonodi**. Lymph node. 2nd declension masc.

M

- **Macula**, pl. **maculae**, gen. **maculae**. Macula, spot. 1st declension fem.
- **Magnus**, pl. **magni**, gen. **magni**. Large, great. 2nd declension masc. (adj.: masc. *magnus*, fem. *magna*, neut. *magnum*)
- **Major**, pl. **majores**, gen. **majoris**. Greater. 3rd declension masc./fem.
- **Malleolus**, pl. **malleoli**, gen. **malleoli**. Malleolus (lit. *small hammer*). 2nd declension masc.
- **Malleus**, pl. **mallei**, gen. **mallei**. Malleus (lit. *hammer*). 2nd declension masc.
- **Mamilla**, pl. **mamillae**, gen. **mamillae**. Mamilla. 1st declension fem.
- **Mamma**, pl. **mammae**, gen. **mammae**. Breast. 1st declension fem.
- **Mandibula**, pl. **mandibulae**, gen. **mandibulae**. Jaw. 1st declension fem.
- **Mandibular**, pl. **mandibulares**, gen. **mandibularis**. Relative to the jaw. 3rd declension.
- **Manubrium**, pl. **manubria**, gen. **manubrii**. Manubrium (lit. *handle*). 2nd declension neut.
  - *Manubrium sterni*, pl. *manubria sterna* (superior part of the sternum)
- **Manus**, pl. **manus**, gen. **manus**. Hand. 4th declension fem.
- **Margo**, pl. **margines**, gen. **marginis**. Margin. 3rd declension fem.
- **Matrix**, pl. **matrices**, gen. **matricis**. Matrix (formative portion of a structure, surrounding substance). 3rd declension fem.
- **Maxilla**, pl. **maxillae**, gen. **maxillae**. Maxilla. 1st declension fem.
- **Maximus**, pl. **maximi**, gen. **maximi**. The greatest, the biggest, the largest. 2nd declension masc. (adj.: masc. *maximus*, fem. *maxima*, neut. *maximum*)

- **Meatus**, pl. **meatus**, gen. **meatus**. Meatus, canal. 4th declension masc.
- **Medialis**, pl. **mediales**, gen. **medialis**. Medial. 3rd declension masc./fem. (adj.: masc. *medialis*, fem. *medialis*, neut. *mediale*)
- **Medium**, pl. **media**, gen. **medii**. Substance, culture medium, means. 2nd declension neut.
- **Medulla**, pl. **medullae**, gen. **medullae**. Marrow. 1st declension fem.
  - *Medulla oblongata* (caudal portion of the brainstem), *medulla spinalis*
- **Membrana**, pl. **membranae**, gen. **membranae**. Membrane. 1st declension fem.
- **Membrum**, pl. **membra**, gen. **membri**. Limb. 2nd declension neut.
- **Meningitis**, pl. **meningitides**, gen. **meningitidis**. Meningitis. 3rd declension fem.
- **Meningococcus**, pl. **meningococci**, gen. **meningococci**. Meningococcus. 2nd declension masc.
- **Meninx**, pl. **meninges**, gen. **meningis**. Meninx. 3rd declension.
- **Meniscus**, pl. **menisci**, gen. **menisci**. Meniscus. 2nd declension masc.
- **Mentum**, pl. **menti**, gen. **menti**. Chin. 2nd declension masc.
- **Mesocardium**, pl. **mesocardia**, gen. **mesocardii**. Mesocardium. 2nd declension neut.
- **Mesothelium**, pl. **mesothelia**, gen. **mesothelii**. Mesothelium. 2nd declension neut.
- **Metacarpus**, pl. **metacarpi**, gen. **metacarpi**. Metacarpus. 2nd declension masc.
- **Metaphysis**, pl. **metaphyses**, gen. **metaphysis**. Metaphysis. 3rd declension.
- **Metastasis**, pl. **metastases**, gen. **metastasis**. Metastasis. 3rd declension
- **Metatarsus**, pl. **metatarsi**, gen. **metatarsi**. Metatarsus. 2nd declension masc.
- **Microvillus**, pl. **microvilli**, gen. **microvilli**. Microvillus (from *villus*, hair). 2nd declension masc.
- **Minimus**, pl. **minimi**, gen. **minimi**. The smallest, the least. 2nd declension masc. (adj.: masc. *minimus*, fem. *minima*, neut. *minimum*)
- **Minor**, pl. **minores**, gen. **minoris**. Lesser. 3rd declension masc.
- **Mitochondrion**, pl. **mitochondria**, gen. **mitochondrium**. Mitochondrion. 3rd declension neut.
- **Mitosis**, pl. **mitoses**, gen. **mitosis**. Mitosis. 3rd declension (from Gr. *mitos*, thread)
- **Mons**, pl. **montes**, gen. **montis**. Mons (lit. *mountain*). 3rd declension masc.
- **Mors**, pl. **mortes**, gen. **mortis**, acc. **mortem**. Death. 3rd declension fem.
- **Mucolipidosis**, pl. **mucolipidoses**, gen. **mucolipidosis**. Mucolipidosis. 3rd declension masc./fem.
- **Mucro**, pl. **mucrones**, gen. **mucronis**. Sharp-tipped structure. 3rd declension masc.
  - *Mucro sterni* (sternal xyphoides)
- **Musculus**, pl. **musculi**, gen. **musculi**. Muscle. 2nd declension masc.

- **Mycelium**, pl. **mycelia**, gen. **mycelii**. Mycelium, mass of hyphae. 2nd declension neut.
- **Mycoplasma**, pl. **mycoplasmata**, gen. **mycoplasmatis**. Mycoplasma. 3rd declension neut.
- **Mylohyoideus m.**, pl. **mylohyoidei**, gen. **mylohyoidei**. 2nd declension masc.
- **Myocardium**, pl. **myocardia**, gen. **myocardii**. Myocardium. 2nd declension neut.
- **Myofibrilla**, pl. **myofibrillae**, gen. **myofibrillae**. Myofibrilla. 1st declension fem.
- **Myrinx**, pl. **myringes**, gen. **myringis**. Eardrum. 3rd declension.

N

- **Naris**, pl. **nares**, gen. **naris**. Nostril. 3rd declension fem.
- **Nasus**, pl. **nasi**, gen. **nasi**. Nose. 2nd declension masc.
- **Navicularis**, pl. **naviculares**, gen. **navicularis**. Ship shaped. 3rd declension masc.
- **Nebula**, pl. **nebulae**, gen. **nebulae**. Mist, cloud (corneal nebula, corneal opacity). 1st declension fem.
- **Neisseria**, pl. **neisseriae**, gen. **neisseriae**. Neisseria. 1st declension fem.
- **Nephritis**, pl. **nephritides**, gen. **nephritidis**. Nephritis 3rd declension.
- **Nervus**, pl. **nervi**, gen. **nervi**. Nerve. 2nd declension masc.
- **Neuritis**, pl. **neuritides**, gen. **neuritidis**. Neuritis. 3rd declension.
- **Neurosis**, pl. **neuroses**, gen. **neurosis**. Neurosis. 3rd declension.
- **Nevus**, pl. **nevi**, gen. **nevi**. Nevus (lit. mole on the body, birthmark). 2nd declension masc.
- **Nidus**, pl. **nidi**, gen. **nidi**. Nidus (lit. *nest*). 2nd declension masc.
- **Nodulus**, pl. **noduli**, gen. **noduli**. Nodule (small node, knot). 2nd declension masc.
- **Nucleolus**, pl. **nucleoli**, gen. **nucleoli**. Nucleolus (small nucleus). 2nd declension masc.
- **Nucleus**, pl. **nuclei**, gen. **nuclei**. Nucleus (central part, core, lit. *inside of a nut*). 2nd declension masc.

O

- **Obliquus**, pl. **obliqui**, gen. **obliqui**. Oblique. 2nd declension masc. (adj.: masc. *obliquus*, fem. *obliqua*, neut. *obliquum*)
- **Occiput**, pl. **occipita**, gen. **occipitis**. Occiput (back of the head). 3rd declension neut.
- **Oculentum**, pl. **oculenta**, gen. **oculenti**. Eye ointment. 2nd declension neut.
- **Oculus**, pl. **oculi**, gen. **oculi**. Eye. 2nd declension masc.
- **Oliva**, pl. **olivae**, gen. **olivae**. Rounded elevation (lit. *olive*). 1st declension fem.
- **Omentum**, pl. **omenta**, gen. **omenti**. Peritoneal fold. 2nd declension neut.

- **Oogonium**, pl. **oogonia**, gen. **oogonii**. Oocyte. 2nd declension neut.
- **Operculum**, pl. **opercula**, gen. **operculi**. Operculum, cover (lit. *lesser lid*). 2nd declension neut.
- **Orbicularis m.**, pl. **orbiculares**, gen. **orbicularis**. Muscle encircling a structure. 3rd declension masc. (adj.: masc. *orbicularis*, fem. *orbicularis*, neut. *orbiculare*)
- **Organum**, pl. **organa**, gen. **organi**. Organ. 2nd declension neut.
- **Orificium**, pl. **orificia**, gen. **orificii**. Opening, orifice. 2nd declension neut.
- **Os**, pl. **ora**, gen. **oris**. Mouth. 3rd declension neut.
  - *Os* + genitive case: *os coccyges* (coccigeal bone), *os ischii* (ischium)
- **Os**, pl. **ossa**, gen. **ossis**. Bone. 3rd declension neut.
- **Ossiculum**, pl. **ossicula**, gen. **ossiculi**. Ossicle, small bone. 2nd declension masc.
- **Ostium**, pl. **ostia**, gen. **ostii**. Opening into a tubular organ, entrance. 2nd declension neut.
- **Ovalis**, pl. **ovales**, gen. **ovalis**. Oval. 3rd declension masc. (adj.: masc. *ovalis*, fem. *ovalis*, neut. *ovale*)
- **Ovarium**, pl. **ovaria**, gen. **ovarii**. Ovary. 2nd declension neut.
- **Ovulum**, pl. **ovula**, gen. **ovuli**. Ovule. 2nd declension neut.

P

- **Palatum**, pl. **palata**, gen. **palati**. Palate. 2nd declension neut.
- **Palma**, pl. **palmae**, gen. **palmae**. Palm. 1st declension fem.
- **Palmaris**, pl. **palmares**, gen. **palmaris**. Relative to the palm of the hand. 3rd declension masc. (adj.: masc. *palmaris*, fem. *palmaris*, neut. *palmare*)
- **Palpebra**, pl. **palpebrae**, gen. **palpebrae**. Eyelid. 1st declension fem.
- **Pancreas**, pl. **pancreates/pancreata**, gen. **pancreatis**. Pancreas. 3rd declension fem./neut.
- **Panniculus**, pl. **panniculi**, gen. **panniculi**. Panniculus (a layer of tissue, from *pannus*, pl. *panni*, cloth). 2nd declension masc.
- **Pannus**, pl. **panni**, gen. **panni**. Pannus (lit. *cloth*). 2nd declension masc.
- **Papilla**, pl. **papillae**, gen. **papillae**. Papilla (lit. *nipple*). 1st declension fem.
- **Paralysis**, pl. **paralyses**, gen. **paralysos/paralysis**. Palsy. 3rd declension fem.
- **Parametrium**, pl. **parametria**, gen. **parametrii**. Parametrium. 2nd declension neut.
- **Paries**, pl. **parietes**, gen. **parietis**. Wall. 3rd declension masc.
- **Pars**, pl. **partes**, gen. **partis**. Part. 3rd declension fem.
- **Patella**, pl. **patellae**, gen. **patellae**. Patella. 1st declension fem.
- **Pectoralis m.**, pl. **pectorales**, gen. **pectoralis**. Pectoralis muscle. 3rd declension masc. (adj.: masc. *pectoralis*, fem. *pectoralis*, neut. *pectorale*)
- **Pectus**, pl. **pectora**, gen. **pectoris**. Chest. 3rd declension neut.
  - *Pectus excavatum, pectus carinatum*

- **Pediculus**, pl. **pediculi**, gen. **pediculi**. 1. Pedicle. 2. Louse. 2nd declension masc.
- **Pedunculus**, pl. **pedunculi**, gen. **pedunculi**. Pedicle. 2nd declension masc.
- **Pelvis**, pl. **pelves**, gen. **pelvis**. Pelvis. 3rd declension fem.
- **Penis**, pl. **penes**, gen. **penis**. Penis. 3rd declension masc.
- **Perforans**, pl. **perforantes**, gen. **perforantis**. Something which pierces a structure. 3rd declension masc.
- **Pericardium**, pl. **pericardia**, gen. **pericardii**. Pericardium. 2nd declension neut.
- **Perimysium**, pl. **perimysia**, gen. **perimysii**. Perimysium (from Gr. *mysia*, muscle). 2nd declension neut.
- **Perineum**, pl. **perinea**, gen. **perinei**. Perineum. 2nd declension neut.
- **Perineurium**, pl. **perineuria**, gen. **perineurii**. Perineurium (from Gr. *neuron*, nerve). 2nd declension neut.
- **Periodontium**, pl. **periodontia**, gen. **periodontii**. Periodontium (from Gr. *odous*, tooth). 2nd declension neut.
- **Perionychium**, pl. **perionychia**, gen. **perionychii**. Perionychium (from Gr. *onyx*, nail). 2nd declension neut.
- **Periosteum**, pl. **periostea**, gen. **periosteii**. Periosteum (from Gr. *osteon*, bone). 2nd declension neut.
- **Periostosis**, pl. **periostoses**, gen. **periostosis**. Periostosis. 3rd declension.
- **Peritoneum**, pl. **peritonea**, gen. **peritonei**. Peritoneum. 2nd declension neut.
- **Peroneus m.**, pl. **peronei**, gen. **peronei**. Peroneal bone. 2nd declension masc.
- **Pes**, pl. **pedes**, gen. **pedis**. Foot. 3rd declension masc.
- **Petechia**, pl. **petechiae**, gen. **petechiae**. Petechiae (tiny hemorrhagic spots). 1st declension fem.
- **Phalanx**, pl. **phalanges**, gen. **phalangis**. Phalanx (long bones of the digits). 3rd declension fem.
  - *Os phalangi*, pl. *ossa phalangium*
- **Phallus**, pl. **phalli**, gen. **phalli**. Phallus, penis. 2nd declension masc.
- **Pharynx**, pl. **pharynges**, gen. **pharyngis**. Pharynx. 3rd declension.
- **Philtrum**, pl. **philtra**, gen. **philtri**. Philtrum. 2nd declension neut.
- **Phimosis**, pl. **phimoses**, gen. **phimosis**. Phimosis. 3rd declension masc.
- **Phlyctena**, pl. **phlyctenae**, gen. **phlyctenae**. Phlyctena (small blister). 1st declension fem.
- **Pia mater**, pl. **piae matres**, gen. **piae matris**. Pia mater (inner meningeal layer of tissue). 1st declension fem. (adj.: masc. *pius*, fem. *pia*, neut. *pium*, tender)
- **Placenta**, pl. **placentae**, gen. **placentae**. Placenta (lit. *cake*). 1st declension fem.
- **Planta**, pl. **plantae**, gen. **plantae**. Plant, sole. 1st declension fem.
- **Plantar**, pl. **plantaria**, gen. **plantaris**. Relating to the sole of the foot. 3rd declension neut.

- **Planum**, pl. **plana**, gen. **plani**. Plane. 2nd declension neut.
- **Platysma m.**, pl. **platysmata**, gen. **platysmatis**. Platysma. 3rd declension neut.
- **Pleura**, pl. **pleurae**, gen. **pleurae**. Pleura. 1st declension fem.
- **Plica**, pl. **plicae**, gen. **plicae**. Fold. 1st declension fem.
- **Pneumoconiosis**, pl. **pneumoconioses**, gen. **pneumoconiosis**. Pneumoconiosis. 3rd declension.
- **Pollex**, pl. **pollices**, gen. **pollicis**. Thumb. 3rd declension masc.
- **Polus**, pl. **poli**, gen. **poli**. Pole. 2nd declension masc.
- **Pons**, pl. **pontes**, gen. **pontis**. Pons (lit. *bridge*). 3rd declension masc.
- **Porta**, pl. **portae**, gen. **portae**. Porta (from Lat. verb *porto*, carry, bring). 1st declension fem.
- **Portio**, pl. **portiones**, gen. **portionis**. Portion. 3rd declension fem.
- **Porus**, pl. **pori**, gen. **pori**. Pore. 2nd declension masc.
- **Posterior**, pl. **posteriores**, gen. **posterioris**. Coming after. 3rd declension.
- **Praeputium**, pl. **praeputia**, gen. **praeputii**. Prepuce, foreskin. 2nd declension neut.
- **Princeps**, pl. **principes**, gen. **principis**. Princeps (first, foremost, leading). 3rd declension masc.
- **Processus**, pl. **processus**, gen. **processus**. Process. 4th declension masc.
- **Profunda**, pl. **profundae**, gen. **profundae**. Deep. 1st declension fem. (adj.: masc. *profundus*, fem. *profunda*, neut. *profundum*)
  - *Vena femoralis profunda*, deep femoral vein
- **Prominentia**, pl. **prominentiae**, gen. **prominentiae**. Prominence. 1st declension fem.
- **Promontorium**, pl. **promontoria**, gen. **promontorii**. Promontorium. 2nd declension neut.
- **Pronator**, pl. **pronatores**, gen. **pronatoris**. A muscle that serves to pronate. 3rd declension masc.
  - *Pronator teres m.*, *pronator quadratus m.*
- **Prophylaxis**, pl. **prophylaxes**, gen. **prophylaxis**. Prophylaxis (from Gr. *prophylasso*, take precaution). 3rd declension.
- **Proprius**, pl. **proprii**, gen. **proprii**. Own. 2nd declension masc. (adj.: masc. *proprius*, fem. *propria*, neut. *proprium*)
- **Prosthesis**, pl. **prostheses**, gen. **prosthesis**. Prosthesis. 3rd declension fem.
- **Psychosis**, pl. **psychoses**, gen. **psychosis**. Psychosis. 3rd declension fem.
- **Ptosis**, pl. **ptoses**, gen. **ptosis**. Ptosis. 3rd declension.
- **Pubes**, pl. **pubes**, gen. **pubis**. Pubis. 3rd declension fem.
- **Pudendum**, pl. **pudenda**, gen. **pudendi**. Relative to the external genitals (lit. *shameful*). 2nd declension neut. (adj.: masc. *pudendus*, fem. *pudenda*, neut. *pudendum*)
- **Puerpera**, pl. **puerperae**, gen. **puerperae**. Puerpera. 1st declension fem.
- **Puerperium**, pl. **puerperia**, gen. **puerperii**. Puerperium. 2nd declension neut.
- **Pulmo**, pl. **pulmones**, gen. **pulmonis**. Lung. 3rd declension masc.

- **Punctata**, pl. **punctatae**, gen. **punctatae**. Pointed. 1st declension fem.
- **Punctum**, pl. **puncta**, gen. **puncti**. Point. 2nd declension neut.
- **Pylorus**, pl. **pylori**, gen. **pylori**. Pylorus. 2nd declension masc.
- **Pyramidalis m.**, pl. **pyramidales**, gen. **pyramidalis**. Pyramidal. 3rd declension masc. (adj.: masc. *pyramidalis*, fem. *pyramidalis*, neut. *pyramidale*)
- **Pyriformis m.**, pl. **pyriformes**, gen. **pyriformis**. Pear-shaped. 3rd declension masc. (adj.: masc. *pyriformis*, fem. *pyriformis*, neut. *pyriforme*)

Q
- **Quadratus**, pl. **quadrati**, gen. **quadrati**. Square. 2nd declension masc. (adj.: masc. *quadratus*, fem. *quadrata*, neut. *quadratum*)
- **Quadrigemina**, pl. **quadrigeminae**, gen. **quadrigeminae**. Fourfold, in four parts. 1st declension fem. (adj.: *quadrigeminus*, fem. *quadrigemina*, neut. *quadrigeminum*)

R
- **Rachis**, pl. Lat. **rachides**, pl. Engl. **rachises**, gen. **rachidis**. Rachis, vertebral column. 3rd declension.
- **Radiatio**, pl. **radiationes**, gen. **radiationis**. Radiation. 3rd declension fem.
- **Radius**, pl. **radii**, gen. **radii**. Radius. 2nd declension masc.
- **Radix**, pl. **radices**, gen. **radicis**. Root, base. 3rd declension fem.
- **Ramus**, pl. **rami**, gen. **rami**. Branch. 2nd declension masc.
- **Receptaculum**, pl. **receptacula**, gen. **receptaculi**. Receptacle, reservoir. 2nd declension neut.
- **Recessus**, pl. **recessus**, gen. **recessus**. Recess. 4th declension masc.
- **Rectus**, pl. **recti**, gen. **recti**. Right, straight (adj.: masc. *rectus*, fem. *recta*, neut. *rectum*)
  - *Rectus abdominis m.*
- **Regio**, pl. **regiones**, gen. **regionis**. Region. 3rd declension fem.
- **Ren**, pl. **renes**, gen. **renis**. Kidney. 3rd declension masc.
- **Rete**, pl. **retia**, gen. **Retis**. Network, net. 3rd declension neut.
  - *Rete mirabilis*
- **Reticulum**, pl. **reticula**, gen. **reticuli**. Reticulum. 2nd declension neut.
- **Retinaculum**, pl. **retinacula**, gen. **retinaculi**. Retinaculum (retaining band or ligament). 2nd declension neut.
- **Rima**, pl. **rimae**, gen. **rima**. Fissure, slit. 1st declension fem.
- **Rostrum**, pl. **rostra**, gen. **rostri**. Rostrum (beak-shaped structure). 2nd declension neut.
- **Rotundum**, pl. **rotunda**, gen. **rotundi**. Round declension (adj.: masc. *rotundus*, fem. *rotunda*, neut. *rotundum*)
  - *Foramen rotundum*, pl. *foramina rotunda*
- **Ruga**, pl. **rugae**, gen. **rugae**. Wrinkle, fold. 1st declension fem.

S

- **Sacculus**, pl. **sacculi**, gen. **sacculi**. Small pouch. 2nd declension masc.
- **Saccus**, pl. **sacci**, gen. **sacci**. Pouch. 2nd declension masc.
- **Sacrum**, pl. **sacra**, gen. **sacri**. Sacral bone (lit. *sacred vessel*). 2nd declension neut.
- **Salpinx**, pl. **salpinges**, gen. **salpingis**. Fallopian tube. 3rd declension.
- **Sartorius m.**, pl. **sartorii**, gen. **sartorii**. Sartorius muscle (tailor's muscle). 2nd declension masc.
- **Scalenus m.**, gen. **scaleni**, pl. **scaleni**. Uneven. 2nd declension masc.
- **Scapula**, pl. **scapulae**, gen. **scapulae**. Scapula, shoulder blade. 1st declension fem.
- **Sclerosis**, pl. **scleroses**, gen. **sclerosis**. Sclerosis. 3rd declension.
- **Scolex**, pl. **scoleces**, gen. **scolecis**. Scolex. 3rd declension.
- **Scotoma**, pl. **scotomata**, gen. **scotomatis**. Scotoma. 3rd declension neut.
- **Scrotum**, pl. **scrota**, gen. **scroti**. Scrotum. 2nd declension neut.
- **Scutulum**, pl. **scutula**, gen. **scutuli**. Scutulum. 2nd declension neut.
- **Scybalum**, pl. **scybala**, gen. **scybali**. Scybalum. 2nd declension neut.
- **Segmentum**, pl. **segmenta**, gen. **segmenti**. Segment. 2nd declension neut.
- **Sella turcica**, pl. **sellae turcicae**, gen. **sellae turcicae**. Turkish chair. 1st declension fem.
- **Semen**, pl. **semina**, gen. **seminis**. Semen. 3rd declension neut.
- **Semimembranosus m.**, pl. **semimembranosi**, gen. **semimembranosi**. 2nd declension masc.
- **Semitendinosus m.**, pl. **semitendinosi**, gen. **semitendinosi**. 2nd declension masc.
- **Sensorium**, pl. **sensoria**, gen. **sensorii**. Sensorium. 2nd declension neut.
- **Sepsis**, pl. **sepses**, gen. **sepsis**. Sepsis. 3rd declension.
- **Septum**, pl. **septa**, gen. **septi**. Septum. 2nd declension neut.
- **Sequela**, pl. **sequelae**, gen. **sequelae**. Sequela. 1st declension fem.
- **Sequestrum**, pl. **sequestra**, gen. **sequestri**. Sequestrum (from sequester, go-between). 2nd declension neut.
- **Serosa**, pl. **serosae**, gen. **serosae**. Serosa. 1st declension fem.
- **Serratus m.**, pl. **serrati**, gen. **serrati**. Serrated, toothed like a saw. 2nd declension masc.
- **Serum**, pl. **sera**, gen. **seri**. Serum (lit. *whey*). 2nd declension neut.
- **Sinciput**, pl. **sincipita**, gen. **sincipitis**. Sinciput. 3rd declension neut.
- **Sinus**, pl. **sinus**, gen. **sinus**. Sinus. 4th declension masc.
- **Soleus m.**, pl. **solei**, gen. **solei**. Soleus. 2nd declension masc.
- **Spatium**, pl. **spatia**, gen. **spatii**. Space. 2nd declension neut.
- **Spectrum**, pl. **spectra**, gen. **spectri**. Spectrum. 2nd declension neut.
- **Sphincter**, pl. Lat. **sphincteres**, pl. Engl. **sphincters**, gen. **sphincteris**. Sphincter. 3rd declension masc.
- **Spiculum**, pl. **spicula**, gen. **spiculi**. Spike (lit. *sting*). 2nd declension neut.
- **Spina**, pl. **spinae**, gen. **spinae**. Spine. 1st declension fem.
- **Splenium**, pl. **splenia**, gen. **splenii**. Splenium. 2nd declension neut.
  – *Splenius capitis/colli m.*

- **Splenunculus,** pl. **splenunculi,** gen. **splenunculi.** Accessory spleen. 2nd declension masc.
- **Sputum,** pl. **sputa,** gen. **sputi.** Sputum. 2nd declension neut.
- **Squama,** pl. **squamae,** gen. **squamae.** Squama (scale, plate-like structure). 1st declension fem.
- **Stapes,** pl. **stapedes,** gen. **stapedis.** Stapes. 3rd declension masc.
- **Staphylococcus,** pl. **staphylococci,** gen. **staphylococci.** Staphylococcus. 2nd declension masc.
- **Stasis,** pl. **stases,** gen. **stasis.** Stasis. 3rd declension masc.
- **Statoconium,** pl. **statoconia,** gen. **statoconii.** Statoconium. 2nd declension neut.
- **Stenosis,** pl. **stenoses,** gen. **stenosis.** Stenosis. 3rd declension.
- **Stereocilium,** pl. **stereocilia,** gen. **stereocilii.** Stereocilium. 2nd declension neut.
- **Sternocleidomastoideus m.,** pl. **sternocleidomastoidei,** gen. **sternocleidomastoidei.** 2nd declension masc.
- **Sternum,** pl. **sterna,** gen. **sterni.** Sternum. 2nd declension neut.
- **Stigma,** pl. **stigmata,** gen. **stigmatis.** Stigma (mark aiding in diagnosis). 3rd declension neut.
- **Stimulus,** pl. **stimuli,** gen. **stimuli.** Stimulus (lit. *spur*). 2nd declension masc.
- **Stoma,** pl. **stomata,** gen. **stomatis.** Stoma, opening, hole. 3rd declension neut.
- **Stratum,** pl. **strata,** gen. **strati.** Stratum. 2nd declension neut.
- **Stria,** pl. **striae,** gen. **striae.** Fluting, channel. 1st declension fem.
- **Stroma,** pl. **stromata,** gen. **stromatis.** Stroma. 3rd declension neut.
- **Struma,** pl. **strumae,** gen. **strumae.** Struma. 1st declension fem.
- **Subiculum,** pl. **subicula,** gen. **subiculi.** Subiculum. 2nd declension neut.
- **Substantia,** pl. **substantiae,** gen. **substantiae.** Substance. 1st declension fem.
- **Sulcus,** pl. **sulci,** gen. **sulci.** Sulcus. 2nd declension masc.
- **Supercilium,** pl. **supercilia,** gen. **supercilii.** Eyebrow. 2nd declension neut.
- **Superficialis,** pl. **superficiales,** gen. **superficialis.** Superficial. 3rd declension masc. (adj.: masc. *superficialis*, fem. *superficialis*, neut. *superficiale*)
- **Superior,** pl. **superiores,** gen. **superioris.** Higher, upper, greater. 3rd declension.
- **Sustentaculum,** pl. **sustentacula,** gen. **sustentaculi.** Sustentaculum. 2nd declension neut.
- **Sutura,** pl. **suturae,** gen. **suturae.** Suture. 1st declension fem.
- **Symphysis,** pl. **symphyses,** gen. **symphysis.** Symphysis. 3rd declension.
- **Synchondrosis,** pl. **synchondroses,** gen. **synchondrosis.** Synchondrosis. 3rd declension.
- **Syncytium,** pl. **syncytia,** gen. **syncytii.** Syncytium. 2nd declension neut.
- **Syndesmosis,** pl. **syndesmoses,** gen. **syndesmosis.** Syndesmosis. 3rd declension.

- **Synechia,** pl. **synechiae,** gen. **synechiae.** Synechia. 1st declension fem.
- **Syrinx,** pl. **syringes,** gen. **syringis.** Syrinx. 3rd declension.

T
- **Talus,** pl. **tali,** gen. **tali.** Talus. 2nd declension masc.
- **Tarsus,** pl. **tarsi,** gen. **tarsi.** Tarsus. 2nd declension masc.
- **Tectum,** pl. **tecta,** gen. **tecti.** Roof. 2nd declension neut.
- **Tegmen,** pl. **tegmina,** gen. **tegminis.** Roof, covering. 3rd declension neut.
- **Tegmentum,** pl. **tegmenta,** gen. **tegmenti.** Covering. 2nd declension neut.
- **Tela,** pl. **telae,** gen. **telae.** Membrane (lit. *web*). 1st declension fem.
- **Telangiectasis,** pl. **telangiectases,** gen. **telangiectasis.** Telangiectasis. 3rd declension.
- **Temporalis m.,** pl. **temporales,** gen. **temporalis.** 3rd declension masc. (adj.: masc. *temporalis,* fem. *temporalis,* neut. *temporale*)
- **Tenaculum,** pl. **tenacula,** gen. **tenaculi.** Surgical clamp. 2nd declension neut.
- **Tendo,** pl. **tendines,** gen. **tendinis.** Tendon, sinew (from verb *tendo,* stretch). 3rd declension masc.
- **Tenia,** pl. **teniae,** gen. **teniae.** Tenia. 1st declension fem.
- **Tensor,** pl. **tensores,** gen. **tensoris.** Something that stretches, that tenses a muscle. 3rd declension masc.
- **Tentorium,** pl. **tentoria,** gen. **tentorii.** Tentorium. 2nd declension neut.
- **Teres,** pl. **teretes,** gen. **teretis.** Round and long. 3rd declension masc.
- **Testis,** pl. **testes,** gen. **testis.** Testicle. 3rd declension masc.
- **Thalamus,** pl. **thalami,** gen. **thalami.** Thalamus (lit. *marriage bed*). 2nd declension masc.
- **Theca,** pl. **thecae,** gen. **thecae.** Theca, envelope (lit. *case, box*). 1st declension fem.
- **Thelium,** pl. **thelia,** gen. **thelii.** Nipple. 2nd declension neut.
- **Thenar,** pl. **thenares,** gen. **thenaris.** Relative to the palm of the hand. 3rd declension neut.
- **Thesis,** pl. **theses,** gen. **thesis.** Thesis. 3rd declension fem.
- **Thorax,** pl. **thoraces,** gen. **thoracos/thoracis.** Chest. 3rd declension masc.
- **Thrombosis,** pl. **thromboses,** gen. **thombosis.** Thrombosis. 3rd declension.
- **Thrombus,** pl. **thrombi,** gen. **thrombi.** Thrombus, clot (from Gr. *thrombos*). 2nd declension masc.
- **Thymus,** pl. **thymi,** gen. **thymi.** Thymus. 2nd declension masc.
- **Tibia,** pl. **tibiae,** gen. **tibiae.** Tibia. 1st declension fem.
- **Tonsilla,** pl. **tonsillae,** gen. **tonsillae.** Tonsil. 1st declension fem.
- **Tophus,** pl. **tophi,** gen. **tophi.** Tophus. 2nd declension masc.
- **Torulus,** pl. **toruli,** gen. **toruli.** Papilla, small elevation. 2nd declension masc.
- **Trabecula,** pl. **trabeculae,** gen. **trabeculae.** Trabecula (supporting bundle of either osseous or fibrous fibers). 1st declension fem.
- **Trachea,** pl. **tracheae,** gen. **tracheae.** Trachea. 1st declension fem.

- **Tractus**, pl. **tractus**, gen. **tractus**. Tract. 4th declension masc.
- **Tragus**, pl. **tragi**, gen. **tragi**. Tragus, hircus. 2nd declension masc.
- **Transversalis**, pl. **transversales**, gen. **transversalis**. Transverse. 3rd declension (adj.: masc. *transversalis*, fem. *transversalis*, neut. *transversale*)
- **Transversus**, pl. **transversi**, gen. **transversi**. Lying across, from side to side. 2nd declension masc. (adj.: masc. *transversus*, fem. *transversa*, neut. *transversum*)
- **Trapezium**, pl. **trapezia**, gen. **trapezii**. Trapezium bone. 2nd declension neut.
- **Trauma**, pl. **traumata**, gen. **traumatis**. Trauma. 3rd declension neut.
- **Triangularis**, pl. **triangulares**, gen. **triangularis**. Triangular. 3rd declension masc. (adj.: masc. *triangularis*, fem. *triangularis*, neut. *triangulare*)
- **Triceps**, pl. **tricipes**, gen. **tricipis**. Triceps (from *ceps*, pl. *cipes*, gen. *cipis*, headed). 3rd declension masc.
- **Trigonum**, pl. **trigona**, gen. **trigoni**. Trigonum (lit. *triangle*). 2nd declension neut.
- **Triquetrum**, pl. **triquetra**, gen. **triquetri**. Triquetrum, triquetral bone, pyramidal bone. 2nd declension neut. (adj.: masc. *triquetrus*, fem. *triquetra*, neut. *triquetrum*. Three-cornered, triangular)
- **Trochlea**, pl. **trochleae**, gen. **trochleae**. Trochlea (lit. *pulley*). 1st declension fem.
- **Truncus**, pl. **trunci**, gen. **trunci**. Trunk. 2nd declension masc.
- **Tuba**, pl. **tubae**, gen. **tubae**. Tube. 1st declension fem.
- **Tuberculum**, pl. **tubercula**, gen. **tuberculi**. Tuberculum, swelling, protuberance. 2nd declension neut.
- **Tubulus**, pl. **tubuli**, gen. **tubuli**. Tubule. 2nd declension masc.
- **Tunica**, pl. **tunicae**, gen. **tunicae**. Tunic. 1st declension fem.
- **Tylosis**, pl. **tyloses**, gen. **tylosis**. Tylosis (callosity). 3rd declension.
- **Tympanum**, pl. **tympana**, gen. **tympani**. Tympanum, eardrum (lit. *small drum*). 2nd declension neut.

U

- **Ulcus**, pl. **ulcera**, gen. **ulceris**. Ulcer. 3rd declension neut.
- **Ulna**, pl. **ulnae**, gen. **ulnae**. Ulna (lit. *forearm*). 1st declension fem.
- **Umbilicus**, pl. **umbilici**, gen. **umbiculi**. Navel. 2nd declension masc.
- **Uncus**, pl. **unci**, gen. **unci**. Uncus (lit. *hook*, *clamp*). 2nd declension masc.
- **Unguis**, pl. **ungues**, gen. **unguis**. Nail, claw. 3rd declension masc.
- **Uterus**, pl. **uteri**, gen. **uteri**. Uterus, womb. 2nd declension masc.
- **Utriculus**, pl. **utriculi**, gen. **utriculi**. Utriculus (lit. *wineskin*). 2nd declension masc.
- **Uveitis**, pl. **uveitides**, gen. **uveitidis**. Uveítis. 3rd declension fem.
- **Uvula**, pl. **uvulae**, gen. **uvulae**. Uvula (lit. *small grape*, from *uva*, pl. *uvae*, grape). 1st declension fem.

V

- **Vagina**, pl. **vaginae**, gen. **vaginae**. Vagina, sheath. 1st declension fem.
- **Vaginitis**, pl. **vaginitides**, gen. **vaginitidis**. Vaginitis. 3rd declension fem.
- **Vagus**, pl. **vagi**, gen. **vagi**. Vagus nerve. 2nd declension masc. (adj.: masc. *vagus*, fem. *vaga*, neut. *vagum*. Roving, wandering)
- **Valva**, pl. **valvae**, gen. **valvae**. Leaflet. 1st declension fem.
- **Valvula**, pl. **valvulae**, gen. **valvulae**. Valve. 1st declension fem.
- **Varix**, pl. **varices**, gen. **varicis**. Varix, varicose vein. 3rd declension masc.
- **Vas**, pl. **vasa**, gen. **vasis**. Vessel. 3rd declension neut.
  - *Vas deferens, vasa recta, vasa vasorum*
- **Vasculum**, pl. **vascula**, gen. **vasculi**. Small vessel. 2nd declension neut.
- **Vastus**, pl. **vasti**, gen. **vasti**. Vast, huge. 2nd declension neut. (adj.: masc. *vastus*, fem. *vasta*, neut. *vasti*)
  - *Vastus medialis/intermedius/lateralis m.*
- **Vasum**, pl. **vasa**, gen. **vasi**. Vessel. 2nd declension neut.
- **Velum**, pl. **veli**, gen. **veli**. Covering, curtain (lit. *sail*). 2nd declension neut.
- **Vena**, pl. **venae**, gen. **venae**. Vein. 1st declension fem.
  - *Vena cava*, pl. *venae cavae*, gen. *venae cavae* (from adj. *cavus/a/um*, hollow)
- **Ventriculus**, pl. **ventriculi**, gen. **ventriculi**. Ventricle (lit. *small belly*). 2nd declension masc.
- **Venula**, pl. **venulae**, gen. **venulae**. Venule. 1st declension fem.
- **Vermis**, pl. **vermes**, gen. **vermis**. Worm. 3rd declension masc.
- **Verruca**, pl. **verrucae**, gen. **verrucae**. Wart. 1st declension fem.
- **Vertebra**, pl. **vertebrae**, gen. **vertebrae**. Vertebra. 1st declension fem.
- **Vertex**, pl. **vertices**, gen. **verticis**. Vertex (lit. *peak, top*). 3rd declension masc.
- **Vesica**, pl. **vesicae**, gen. **vesicae**. Bladder. 1st declension fem.
- **Vesicula**, pl. **vesiculae**, gen. **vesiculae**. Vesicle (lit. *lesser bladder*). 1st declension fem.
- **Vestibulum**, pl. **vestibula**, gen. **vestibuli**. Entrance to a cavity. 2nd declension neut.
- **Villus**, pl. **villi**, gen. **villi**. Villus (shaggy hair). 2nd declension masc.
- **Vinculum**, pl. **vincula**, gen. **vinculi**. Band, band-like structure (lit. *chain, bond*). 2nd declension neut.
- **Virus**, pl. Lat. **viri**, pl. Engl. **viruses**, gen. **viri**. Virus. 2nd declension masc.
- **Viscus**, pl. **viscera**, gen. **visceris**. Viscus, internal organ. 3rd declension neut.
- **Vitiligo**, pl. **vitiligines**, gen. **vitiligis**. Vitiligo. 3rd declension masc.
- **Vomer**, pl. **vomeres**, gen. **vomeris**. Vomer bone. 3rd declension masc.
- **Vulva**, pl. **vulvae**, gen. **vulvae**. Vulva. 1st declension fem.

Z

- **Zona,** pl. **zonae,** gen. **zonae.** Zone. 1st declension fem.
- **Zonula,** pl. **zonulae,** gen. **zonulae.** Small zone. 1st declension fem.
- **Zygapophysis,** pl. **zygapophyses,** gen. **zygapophysis.** Vertebral articular apophysis. 3rd declension fem.

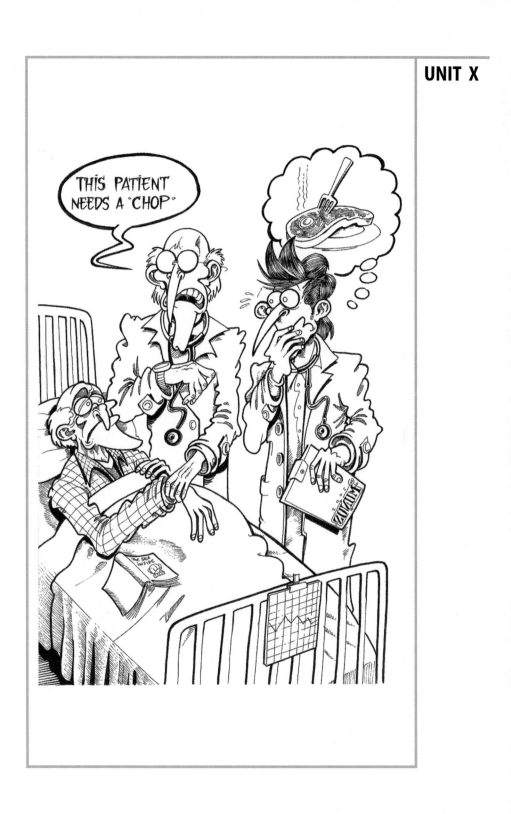

Unit X   Acronyms and Abbreviations

Introduction

"The patient went from the ER to the OR and then to the ICU." It is an irrefutable fact that doctor's speech is full of abbreviations. Health-care professionals in general and cardiologists in particular use many abbreviations. This high prevalence has led us to consider medical abbreviations as a challenging pandemic.

There are several "types" of abbreviations, namely:
- Straightforward abbreviations
- Extra-nice abbreviations
- Expanded-term abbreviations
- Energy-saving abbreviations
- Double-meaning abbreviations
- Mind-blowing abbreviations

Let us begin with the nice ones; we call them the straightforward abbreviations because for each nice abbreviation in your own language there is a nice English equivalent. No beating around the bush here; it is just a matter of changing letter order, identifying the abbreviations and learning them. Let us give you a few examples so you can enjoy the simple things in life ... while you can!

HRT   Hormone-replacement therapy
LVOT   Left ventricle outflow tract
ASD   Atrial septal defect
VSD   Ventricular septal defect
TEE   Transesophageal echocardiography
LAD   Left anterior descending artery
ACE   Angiotensin-converting enzyme

There are other kinds of abbreviations: the *extra-nice* ones. They are mostly used for drugs or chemical substances whose name has three or four syllables too many. They are extra nice because they are usually the same in many languages. Let us see just an example:

CPK   Creatine phosphokinase

In the next group, we have put together some examples of abbreviations that are widely used in English but that are generally preferred in their expanded form in other languages. Since language is an ever-changing creature, we are sure that these terms will eventually be abbreviated in many languages but so far you hear them referred to mostly as expanded terms:

PBSC   Peripheral blood stem cell
AVNRT   Atrioventricular nodal reentrant tachycardia

There is another group, which we call the energy-saving abbreviations. These are abbreviations that many languages leave in the English original and, of course, when expanding them the first letter of each word does not match the abbreviation. We call them energy saving because it would not have been so difficult to come up with a real "national" abbreviation for that term. When looking for examples, we realized that most hormone names are energy-saving abbreviations:

FSH   Follicle-stimulating hormone
TNF   Tumor necrosis factor
PAWP   Pulmonary arterial wedge pressure

There is yet another kind, which we call the double-meaning abbreviations. This is when one abbreviation can refer to two different terms. The context helps, of course, to discern the real meaning. However, it is worth keeping an eye open for these because, if misinterpreted, these abbreviations might get you into an embarrassing situation:

- AED
  - Automatic external defibrillator
  - Anti-epileptic drug
- BE
  - Bacterial endocarditis
  - Barium enema
- BS
  - Bowel sounds
  - Breath sounds
  - Blood sugar
- HSM
  - Holosystolic murmur
  - Hepatosplenomegaly

- PT
  - Physical therapy
  - Posterior tibial
  - Prothrombin time
  - Patient
- RAD
  - Right axis deviation
  - Reactive airways disease

The funniest abbreviations are those that become acronyms in which the pronunciation resembles a word that has nothing to do with the abbreviation's meaning. We call this group the mind-blowing abbreviations.

A "cabbage" in English is that nice vegetable known for its gasogenic properties. However, when an English-speaking cardiologist says "This patient is a clear candidate for cabbage," he/she isn't talking about what the patient should have for lunch, but rather the type of surgery he/she is suggesting should be performed. Thus, "cabbage" is the colloquial way of referring to CABG (coronary artery bypass grafting).

There are more abbreviations out there, and there are more to come. The medical profession is sure to keep us busy catching up with its incursions into linguistic creation.

Regardless of the "type" of abbreviation you have before you, we will give you three pieces of advice:

1. Identify the most common abbreviations.
2. Read the abbreviations in your lists.
3. Begin with abbreviation lists of your cardiologic subspecialty.

Read the abbreviations in your lists. Read the abbreviations in your lists in a natural way. Bear in mind that to be able to identify written abbreviations may not be enough. From this standpoint, there are three types of abbreviations:

1. Spelled abbreviations
2. Read abbreviations (acronyms)
3. Half-spelled/half-read abbreviations

Nobody would understand a spelled abbreviation if you read it, and nobody would understand a read abbreviation if you spelled it. Let us make clear what we are trying to say with an example. "LIMA" stands for left internal mammary artery and must be read *lima*. Nobody would understand you if instead of saying *lima* you spell L-I-M-A. Therefore, never spell a "read abbreviation" and never read a "spelled abbreviation."

Most abbreviations are spelled abbreviations, and are usually those in which the letter order makes them almost impossible to read. Think, for example, of COPD (chronic obstructive pulmonary disease) and try to read the abbreviation instead of spelling it. Never use the "expanded form" (chronic obstructive pulmonary disease) of a classic abbreviation such as this one, because it would sound extraordinarily unnatural.

Some abbreviations have become acronyms and therefore must be read and not spelled. Their letter order allows us to read them. LIMA belongs to this group.

The third type is made up of abbreviations such as CPAP (continuous positive airway pressure) which is pronounced something like *C-pap*. If you spell out CPAP (C-P-A-P), nobody will understand you.

Review abbreviation lists on your specialty. Review as many abbreviation lists on your specialty as you can and double-check them until you are familiar with their meaning and pronunciation.

Although you should make your own abbreviation lists, we have created several classified by specialty. To begin with, check whether your own specialty's list is included; if not, start writing your own. Be patient; this task can last the rest of your professional life.

Abbreviation Lists

Oriented General List

AA	Alcoholics Anonymous; African American
A-a	Alveolar arterial gradient
AAA	Abdominal aortic aneurysm
AB	Antibody; also abortion
ABD	Abdomen
ABG	Arterial blood gas
ABI	Ankle-brachial index
ABPA	Allergic bronchopulmonary aspergillosis
ABX	Antibiotics
AC	Anterior chamber; also acromioclavicular, and before meals (a.c.)
ACE-I	Angiotensin-converting enzyme inhibitor
ACL	Anterior cruciate ligament
ACLS	Advanced cardiac life support
ACS	Acute coronary syndrome
AD LIB	As desired
ADA	American Diabetes Association
ADD	Attention deficit disorder
ADE	Adverse drug effect
ADHD	Attention deficit hyperactivity disorder
ADL	Activities of daily living
ADR	Adverse drug reaction
ADTP	Alcohol and drug treatment program

AED	Automatic external defibrillator; anti-epileptic drug
AF	Atrial fibrillation; also afebrile
AFB	Acid-fast bacterium
AFP	Alpha fetoprotein
AGN	Antigen
AI	Aortic insufficiency
AIDS	Acquired immunodeficiency syndrome
AIN	Acute interstitial nephritis
AK	Actinic keratosis
AKA	Above-knee amputation
ALL	Allergies; also acute lymphocytic leukemia
ALS	Amyotrophic lateral sclerosis; also advanced life support
AMA	Against medical advice; American Medical Association
AMD	Aging macular degeneration
AMI	Acute myocardial infarction; anterior myocardial infarction
A-MIBI	Adenosine MIBI
AML	Acute myelogenous leukemia
AMS	Altered mental status; acute mountain sickness
ANC	Absolute neutrophil count
AND	Axillary node dissection
ANGIO	Angiography
A&O	Alert and oriented
AP	Anterior-posterior
A/P	Assessment and plan
APC	Atrial premature contraction
APD	Afferent pupillary defect
APPY	Appendectomy
APS	Adult protective services
ARB	Angiotensin-receptor blocker
ARDS	Adult respiratory distress syndrome
ARF	Acute renal failure
AS	Aortic stenosis; also ankylosing spondylitis
ASA	Aspirin
ASD	Atrial septal defect
ASU	Ambulatory surgery unit
ATN	Acute tubular necrosis
A/V nicking	Arteriolar/venous nicking
A/V ratio	Arteriolar/venous ratio
AVF	Arteriovenous fistula
AVM	Arterial venous malformation
AVN	Avascular necrosis; atrioventricular
AVNRT	Atrioventricular nodal re-entrant tachycardia
AVR	Aortic valve replacement
AVSS	Afebrile, vital signs stable

B	Bilateral
B&C	Board and care
BAE	Barium enema
BBB	Bundle branch block
BCC	Basal cell carcinoma
BCG	Bacille Calmette-Guérin (vaccine)
BDR	Background diabetic retinopathy
BE	Bacterial endocarditis; also barium enema
BET	Benign essential tremor
BIB	Brought in by
BID	Twice a day
BIPAP	Bi-level positive airway pressure
BIVAD	Bi-ventricular assist device
BKA	Below-knee amputation
BL CX	Blood culture
BM	Bone marrow; also bowel movement
BMI	Body mass index
BMT	Bone marrow transplant
BP	Blood pressure
BPD	Borderline personality disorder; also bipolar disorder and bronchopulmonary dysplasia
BPV	Benign positional vertigo
BR	Bed rest
BRAO	Branch retinal artery occlusion
BRB	Bright red blood
BRBPR	Bright red blood per rectum
BRP	Bathroom privileges
BRVO	Branch retinal vein occlusion
BS	Bowel sounds; also breath sounds, and blood sugar
BSA	Body surface area
BUN	Blood urea nitrogen
BX	Biopsy
c̄	With
CABG	Coronary artery bypass graft
CAD	Coronary artery disease
CAP	Prostate cancer; community-acquired pneumonia
CARDS	Cardiology
CAT	Cataract
CATH	Catheterization
CB	Cerebellar
C/B	Complicated by
CBC	Complete blood count
CBD	Common bile duct; closed-bag drainage
CBI	Continuous bladder irrigation
CC	Chief complaint

CCB	Calcium channel blocker
CCC	Central corneal clouding
CCK	Cholecystectomy
CCE	Clubbing, cyanosis, edema
C/D	Cup-to-disk ratio
CDI	Clean, dry, and intact
C DIF	*Clostridium difficile*
CEA	Carcinoembryonic antigen
Chemo	Chemotherapy
CHI	Closed head injury
CHF	Congestive heart failure
Chole	Cholecystectomy
CI	Cardiac index
CIC	Clean intermittent catheterization
CIDP	Chronic inflammatory demyelinating polyneuropathy
CK	Creatinine kinase
CL	Chloride
CLL	Chronic lymphocytic leukemia
CM	Cardiomegaly
CML	Chronic myelogenous leukemia
CMP	Cardiomyo pathy
CMR	Chief medical resident
CMT	Cervical Motion Tenderness; Charcot-Marie-Tooth (disease)
CMV	Cytomegalo virus
CN	Cranial nerves
CNIS	Carotid non-invasive study
CNS	Central nervous system
CO	Cardiac output
C/O	Complains of
COPD	Chronic obstructive pulmonary disease
COX 2	Cyclooxygenase 2
CPAP	Continuous positive airway pressure
CPP	Cerebral perfusion pressure
CPPD	Calcium pyrophosphate disease
CPR	Cardiopulmonary resuscitation
CPS	Child protective services
CPU	Chest pain unit
CRAO	Central retinal artery occlusion
CRFs	Cardiac risk factors
CRI	Chronic renal insufficiency
CRP	C-reactive protein
CRVO	Central retinal vein occlusion
CSF	Cerebral spinal fluid
CT	Cat scan; also chest tube, and cardiothoracic
CTA	Clear to auscultation
CVA	Cerebral vascular accident

CVL	Central venous line
CVP	Central venous pressure
C/W	Consistent with; compared with
CX	Culture
CXR	Chest X-ray
C/W	Consistent with
D	Diarrhea; also disk
D5W	Dextrose 5% in water
DB	Direct bilirubin
DBP	Diastolic blood pressure
DC	Discharge; discontinue; doctor of chiropractics
D&C	Dilatation and curettage
DCIS	Ductal carcinoma in situ
DDX	Differential diagnosis
DF	Dorsiflexion
DFA	Direct fluorescent antibody
DFE	Dilated fundus examination
DI	Diabetes insipidus; detrusor instability
DIC	Disseminated intravascular coagulopathy
DIF	Differential
DIP	Distal interphalangeal
DJD	Degenerative joint disease
DKA	Diabetic ketoacidosis
DM	Diabetes mellitus
DNI	Do not intubate
DNR	Do not resuscitate
DO	Doctor of osteopathy
D/O	Disorder
DOT	Directly observed therapy
DOU	Direct observation unit
DP	Dorsalis pedis
DPL	Diagnostic peritoneal lavage
DPOA	Durable power of attorney
DR	Diabetic retinopathy
DRE	Digital rectal exam
D/T	Due to
DTs	Delirium tremens
DTR	Deep tendon reflex
DVT	Deep venous thrombosis
DX	Diagnosis
DU	Duodenal ulcer
EBL	Estimated blood loss
EBM	Evidence-based medicine
EBRT	External-beam radiation therapy

EBV	Epstein-Barr virus
ECG	Electrocardiogram (also known as EKG)
ECHO	Echocardiography
ECMO	Extracorporeal membrane oxygenation
ECT	Electroconvulsive therapy
ED	Erectile dysfunction
EEG	Electroencephalogram
EF	Ejection fraction (in reference to ventricular function)
EGD	Esophagogastroduodenoscopy
EIC	Epidermal inclusion cyst
EJ	External jugular
EKG	Electrocardiogram (also known as ECG)
EM	Electron microscopy
EMG	Electromyelogram
EMS	Emergency medical system
EMT	Emergency medical technician
E/O	Evidence of
EOMI	Extraocular muscles intact
Eos	Eosinophils
EPO	Erythropoietin
EPS	Electrophysiologic Study
ER	External rotation; also emergency room
ERCP	Endoscopic retrograde cholangiopancreatography
ES	Epidural steroids
ESI	Epidural steroid injection
ESLD	End-stage liver disease
ESR	Erythrocyte sedimentation rate
ESRD	End-stage renal disease
ESWL	Extracorporeal shock wave lithotripsy
ETOH	Alcohol
ETT	Exercise tolerance test; also endotracheal tube
EWCL	Extended-wear contact lens
EX LAP	Exploratory laparotomy
EX FIX	External fixation
EXT	Extremities
FB	Foreign body
F/B	Followed by
FBS	Fasting blood sugar
FE	Iron
FEM	Femoral
FENA	Fractional excretion of sodium
FEV_1	Forced expiratory volume 1 second
FFP	Fresh frozen plasma
Flex Sig	Flexible sigmoidoscopy
FLU	Influenza

FMG	Foreign medical graduate
F&N	Febrile and neutropenic
FNA	Fine-needle aspiration
FOOSH	Fall on outstretched hand
FOS	Full of stool; force of stream
FP	Family practitioner
FRC	Functional residual capacity
FSG	Finger-stick glucose
FSH	Follicle-stimulating hormone
FTT	Failure to thrive
F/U	Follow-up
FUO	Fever of unknown origin
FX	Fracture
G	Guaiac (followed by + or –)
GA	General anesthesia
GAD	Generalized anxiety disorder
GAS	Group A strep; guaiac all stools
GB	Gall bladder; also Guillain-Barré
GBM	Glioblastoma multiforme
GBS	Group B strep
GC	Gonorrhea
GCS	Glasgow Coma Scale
GCSF	Granulocyte colony-stimulating factor
GERD	Gastroesophageal reflux
GERI	Geriatrics
GET	General endotracheal
GI	Gastrointestinal
GIB	Gastrointestinal bleeding
GLC	Glaucoma
GMR	Gallup, murmurs, rubs
GN	Glomerulonephritis
GNR	Gram-negative rod
GOO	Gastric outlet obstruction
GP	General practitioner
G#P#	Gravida no./Para no.
GP 2b/3a	Glycoprotein 2b/3a Inhibitor
GPC	Gram-positive coccus
GS	Gram stain
GSW	Gunshot wound
GTT	Glucose-tolerance test
G-tube	Gastric feeding tube
GU	Genitourin ary; also gastric ulcer
GVHD	Graft-versus-host disease

H FLU	Haemophilus influenza
HA	Headache
HAART	Highly active anti-retroviral therapy
HACE	High-altitude cerebral edema
HAPE	High-altitude pulmonary edema
H2	Histamine 2
HCC	Hepatocellular carcinoma
HCG	Human chorionic gonadotropin
HCL	Hard contact lens
HCM	Health care maintenance
HCT	Hematocrit
HCV	Hepatitis C virus
HD	Hemodialysis
HDL	High-density lipoprotein
HEENT	Head, ears, eyes, nose, throat
HELLP	Hemolysis-elevated liver tests low platelets
HEME/ONC	Hematology/oncology
HGB	Hemoglobin
HH	Hiatal hernia
H&H	Hemoglobin and hematocrit
HI	Homicidal ideation
HIB	Haemophilus influenza B vaccine
HIT	Heparin-induced thrombocytopenia
HIV	Human immunodeficiency virus
HL	Heparin lock
HOB	Head of bed
HOCM	Hypertrophic obstructive cardiomyopathy
HOH	Hard of hearing
HONK	Hyperosmolar non-ketotic state
HPI	History of present illness
HPV	Human papilloma virus
HR	Heart rate
HRT	Hormone-replacement therapy
HS	At bedtime
HSM	Holosystolic murmur; also hepatosplenomegaly
HSP	Henoch-Schonlein purpura
HSV	Herpes simplex virus
HTN	Hypertens ion
HU	Holding unit
HUS	Hemolytic uremic syndrome
HX	History
I^+	With ionic contrast (in reference to a CAT scan)
I^-	Without ionic contrast (in reference to a CAT scan)
IA	Intra-articular
IABP	Intra-aortic balloon pump

IBD	Inflammatory bowel disease
IBS	Irritable bowel syndrome
IBW	Ideal body weight
ICD	Implantable cardiac defibrillator
ICH	Intracranial hemorrhage
ICP	Intracranial pressure
ID	Infectious diseases
I&D	Incise and drain
IDDM	Insulin-dependent diabetes mellitus
IFN	Interferon
IH	Inguinal hernia (usually preceded by L or R)
IJ	Internal jugular
IL	Interleukin; indirect laryngoscopy
ILD	Interstitial lung disease
IM	Intramuscular also intramedullary
IMI	Inferior myocardial infarction
IMP	Impression
INR	International normalized ratio
I&O	Ins and outs
IOL	Intraocular lens
IOP	Intraocular pressure
IP	Interphalangeal
IPF	Idiopathic pulmonary fibrosis
IR	Interventional radiology; internal rotation
IRB	Indications, risks, benefits; institutional review board
IT	Intrathecal; information technology
ITP	Idiopathic thrombocytopenia
IUD	Intrauterine device
IUP	Intrauterine pregnancy
IV	Intravenous
IVC	Inferior vena cava
IVDU	Intravenous drug use
IVF	Intravenous fluids; also in vitro fertilization
IVP	Intravenous pyelogram
JP	Jackson-Pratt (drain)
J-tube	Jejunal feeding tube
JVD	Jugular venous distention
JVP	Jugular venous pressure
K^+	Potassium
kcal	Kilocalories
KUB	Kidneys, ureters, and bladder
KVO	Keep vein open

L	Left
LA	Left atrium
LAC	Laceration
LAD	Left anterior descending (coronary artery); left axis deviation
LAP	Laparoscopic; also laparotomy
LAR	Low anterior resection
LBBB	Left bundle branch block
LBO	Large bowel obstruction
LBP	Low back pain
LCL	Lateral collateral ligament
LCX	Left circumflex (coronary artery)
L&D	Labor and delivery
LDH	Lactate dehydrogenase
LDL	Low-density lipoprotein
LE	Lower extremity (usually preceded by R or L); leukocyte esterase
LENIS	Lower extremity non-invasive study
LFT	Liver function test
LH	Luteinizing hormone; left handed; light headed
LHC	Left heart cath
LHRH	Luteinizing hormone-releasing hormone
LIMA	Left internal mammary artery
LLE	Left lower extremity
LLL	Left lower lobe; left lower lid
LLQ	Left lower quadrant
LM	Left main coronary artery
LMA	Laryngeal mask airway
LMD	Local medical doctor
LMN	Lower motor neuron
LMP	Last menstrual period
LN	Lymph node; also liquid nitrogen
LND	Lymph node dissection
LOA	Lysis of adhesions
LOC	Loss of consciousness
LP	Lumbar puncture
LPN	Licensed practical nurse
LR	Lactated ringers
LS	Lumbosacral
LT	Light touch
LUE	Left upper extremity
LUL	Left upper lobe; also left upper lid
LUTS	Lower urinary tract symptoms
LUQ	Left upper quadrant
LV FXN	Left ventricular function
LVAD	Left ventricular assist device

LVEDP	Left ventricular end diastolic pressure
LVH	Left ventricular hypertrophy
LVN	Licensed vocational nurse
LMWH	Low-molecular-weight heparin
LYTES	Electrolytes
MAC	Monitored anesthesia care
MCL	Medial collateral ligament
MCP	Metacarpal-phalangeal
MCV	Mean corpuscular volume
MDRTB	Multidrug-resistant tuberculosis
MEDS	Medicines
MFM	Maternal-fetal medicine
MI	Myocardial infarction
MICU	Medical intensive care unit
MIDCAB	Minimally invasive direct coronary artery bypass
MM	Multiple myeloma
M&M	Morbidity and mortality
MMP	Multiple medical problems
MMR	Measles, mumps, and rubella (vaccine)
MOM	Milk of Magnesia
MR	Mitral regurgitation
MRCP	Magnetic resonance cholangiopancreatography
MRI	Magnetic resonance imaging
MRSA	Methicillin-resistant *Staphylococcus aureus*
MS	Mental status; also mitral stenosis, multiple sclerosis, and morphine sulfate
MSSA	Methicillin-sensitive *Staphylococcus aureus*
MTP	Metatarsal-phalangeal
MVP	Mitral valve prolapse
MVR	Mitral valve replacement
N	Nausea
NA	Not available; also sodium (Na^+)
NAD	No apparent distress; no acute disease
NABS	Normal active bowel sounds
NCAT	Normocephalic atraumatic
NCS	Nerve conduction study
NEB	Nebulizer
NGT	Nasogastric tube
NGU	Non-gonococcal urethritis
NH	Nursing home
NHL	Non-Hodgkin's lymphoma
NICU	Neonatal intensive care unit
NIDDM	Non-insulin dependent diabetes mellitus
NIF	Negative inspiratory force

NKDA	No known drug allergies
NMS	Neuroleptic malignant syndrome
NOS	Not otherwise specified
NP	Nurse practitioner
NPO	Nothing by mouth
NS	Normal saline
NSBGP	Non-specific bowel gas pattern
NSCLC	Non-small cell lung cancer
NSR	Normal sinus rhythm
NT	Nontender
NTD	Nothing to do
NUCS	Nuclear medicine
NYHA	New York Heart Association
OA	Osteoarthritis
OB	Occult blood (followed by + or −)
OCD	Obsessive-compulsive disorder
OCP	Oral contraceptive pill
OD	Right eye
OE	Otitis externa
OLT	Orthotopic liver transplant
OM	Otitis media
ON	Optic nerve; overnight
OOB	Out of bed
OP	Opening pressure
O/P	Oropharynx
O&P	Ovum and parasites
ORIF	Open reduction with internal fixation
ORL	Oto-rhinolaryngology
OS	Left eye
OSA	Obstructive sleep apnea
OT	Occupational therapy
OTC	Over the counter
OTD	Out the door
OU	Both eyes
O/W	Otherwise
P	Pulse
P	Pending
P	After
PA	Posterior-anterior; also physician's assistant
PACU	Post-anesthesia care unit
PAD	Peripheral arterial disease
PALS	Pediatric advanced life support
PBC	Primary billiary cirrhosis
PC/p.c.	After meals

PCA	Patient-controlled analgesia
PCI	Percutaneous coronary intervention
PCKD	Polycystic kidney disease
PCL	Posterior cruciate ligament
PCM	Pacemaker
PCOD	Polycystic ovarian disease
PCP	Primary care physician; also pneumocystis pneumonia
PCR	Polymerase chain reaction
PCWP	Pulmonary capillary wedge pressure
PD	Parkinson's disease; also personality disorder, and peritoneal dialysis
PDA	Patent ductus arteriosus
PE	Physical exam; also pulmonary embolism
PEG	Percutaneous endoscopic gastrostomy
PERRL	Pupils equal, round, reactive to light
PET	Positron emission tomography
PF	Peak flow; also plantar flexion
PFO	Patent foramen ovale
PFTs	Pulmonary function tests
PH	Pinhole
PICC	Peripherally inserted central catheter
PICU	Pediatric intensive care unit
PID	Pelvic inflammatory disease
PIH	Pregnancy-induced hypertension
PIP	Proximal Interphalangeal
PLT	Platelets
PMD	Primary medical doctor
PMH	Past medical history
PMI	Point of maximum impulse
PMN	Polymorphonuclear leukocytes
PMRS	Physical medicine and rehabilitation service
PN	Progress note
PNA	Pneumonia
PNBX	Prostate needle biopsy
PND	Paroxysmal nocturnal dyspnea; also post-nasal drip
PNS	Peripheral nervous system
PO	By mouth
POP	Popliteal
PP	Pin prick
PPD	Purified protein derivative
PPH	Primary pulmonary hypertension
PPI	Proton pump inhibitor
PPN	Peripheral parenteral nutrition
PPTL	Postpartum tubal ligation
PR	Per rectum
PRBCs	Packed red blood cells

PRN	Refers to treatments which patient can receive on an "as-needed" basis
PSA	Prostate-specific antigen
PSC	Primary sclerosing cholangitis
PSH	Past surgical history
PT	Physical therapy; posterior tibial; prothrombin time; patient
PTA	Prior to admission; peritonsilar abscess
PTCA	Percutaneous transluminal coronary angioplasty
P-Thal	Persantine Thallium
PTSD	Post-traumatic stress disorder
PTT	Partial thromboplastin time
PTX	Pneumothorax
PUD	Peptic ulcer disease
PV	Polycythemia vera; portal vein
P VAX	Pneumococcal vaccination
PVC	Premature ventricular contraction
PVD	Peripheral vascular disease; posterior vitreous detachment
PVR	Post void residual
Q/q	Every (refers to a time interval e.g., if followed by 6 (Q6), or q6), means "every 6 hours"; if followed by AM, D, W, or M, means "every morning, day, week, or month," respectively
QHS/q.h.s.	Every night
QID	Four times per day
QNS	Quantity not sufficient
QOD/q.o.d.	Every other day
R	Right
RA	Right atrium
RAD	Right axis deviation; also reactive airway disease
R/B	Referred by; relieved by
RBBB	Right bundle branch block
RBC	Red blood cell
RCA	Right coronary artery
RCC	Renal cell cancer
RCT	Randomized controlled trial; rotator cuff tear
RD	Retinal detachment; also registered dietician
RDI	Respiratory disturbance index
RF	Rheumatoid factor; also risk factor
RFA	Radio frequency ablation; right femoral artery
RHC	Right heart cath
RHD	Rheumatic heart disease
Rheum	Rheumatology
R/I	Rule in
RIG	Rabies immunoglobulin
RIMA	Right internal mammary artery

RLE	Right lower extremity
RLL	Right lower lobe; also right lower lid
RLQ	Right lower quadrant
RML	Right middle lobe
RNEF	Radionuc lide ejection fraction
R/O	Rule out
ROM	Range of motion
ROMI	Rule out myocardial infarction
ROS	Review of systems
RPGN	Rapidly progressive glomerulonephritis
RPLND	Retroperitoneal lymph node dissection
RPR	Rapid plasma reagin
RR	Respiratory rate
RRP	Radical retropubic prostatectomy
RRR	Regular rate and rhythm
RSD	Reflex sympathetic dystrophy
RSV	Respiratory syncytial virus
RT	Respiratory therapy
RTC	Return to clinic
RUE	Right upper extremity
RUG	Retrograde urethrogram
RUL	Right upper lobe; right upper lid
RUQ	Right upper quadrant
RV	Right ventricle; residual volume
RVAD	Right ventricular assist device
RVG	Right ventriculogram
RVR	Rapid ventricular response
Rx	Treatment
$\bar{s}$	Without
2°	Secondary to
SA	Sinoatrial; *Staphylococcus aureus*
SAAG	Serum ascites albumin gradient
SAB	Spontaneous abortion
SAH	Subarachnoid hemorrhage
SBE	Subacute bacterial endocarditis
SBO	Small bowel obstruction
SBP	Spontaneous bacterial peritonitis; systolic blood pressure
SC	Subcutaneous
SCCA	Squamous cell cancer
SCL	Soft contact lens
SCLCA	Small cell lung cancer
SEM	Systolic ejection murmur (with reference to cardiac exam)
SFA	Superficial femoral artery
SFV	Superficial femoral vein
SI	Suicidal ideation

SIADH	Syndrome of inappropriate anti-diuretic hormone secretion
SICU	Surgical intensive care unit
SIDS	Sudden infant death syndrome
SIRS	Systemic inflammatory response syndrome
SK	Seborrheic keratosis; also streptokinase
SL	Sublingual
SLE	Systemic lupus erythematosus; also slit lamp exam
SLR	Straight-leg raise
SNF	Skilled nursing facility
S/P	Status Post; also suprapubic
SPEP	Serum protein electropheresis
SPF	Sun-protection formula
SQ	Subcutaneous
SSI	Sliding scale insulin
SSRI	Selective serotonin reuptake inhibitor
STAT	Immediately
STD	Sexually transmitted disease
STS	Soft tissue swelling
STX	Stricture
SVC	Superior vena cava
SVG	Saphenous vein graft
SW	Social work; stab wound
SX	Symptoms
SZR	Seizure
T	Temperature
T&A	Tonsillectomy and adenoidectomy
TAA	Thoracic aortic aneurysm
TAB	Threatened abortion; also therapeutic abortion
TAH	Total abdominal hysterectomy
TB	Tuberculosis; total bilirubin
T&C	Type and cross
TCA	Tricyclic antidepressant
TC	Current temperature
TCC	Transitional cell cancer
TD	Tetanus and diphtheria vaccination; tardive dyskinesia
TDWBAT	Touch-down weight bearing as tolerated
TEE	Transesophageal echocardiogram
TFs	Tube feeds
TG	Triglycerides
THA	Total hip arthroplasty
THR	Total hip replacement
TIA	Transient ischemic attack
TIBC	Total iron-binding capacity
TID/t.i.d.	Three times per day
TIPS	Transvenous intrahepatic portosystemic shunt

TKA	Total knee arthroplasty
TKR	Total knee replacement
TLC	Triple-lumen catheter; total lung capacity
TM	Tympanic membrane; maximum temperature
TMJ	Temporomandibular joint
TMN	Tumor metastases nodes (universal tumor staging system)
TNF	Tumor necrosis factor
TOA	Tubo-ovarian abscess
TOX	Toxicology
TOXO	Toxoplasmosis
TP	Total protein
TPA	Tissue plasminogen activator
TPN	Total parenteral nutrition
TR	Tricuspid regurgitation
TRUS	Transrectal ultrasound
T&S	Type and screen
TSH	Thyroid-stimulating hormone
TTE	Transthor acic echocardiogram
TTP	Tender to palpation; thrombotic thrombocytopenic purpura
TURBT	Transurethral resection bladder tumor
TURP	Transurethral prostatectomy
TV	Tidal volume
TVC	True vocal cord
Tx	Transfusion; treatment
UA	Urine analysis; also uric acid
UC	Ulcerative colitis
UCC	Urgent care center
UCX	Urine culture
UDS	Urodynamic study
UE	Upper extremity (usually preceded by R or L)
UF	Ultrafiltration
UFH	Unfractionated heparin
UMBO	Umbilical
UMN	Upper motor neuron
UNSA	Unstable angina
UO	Urine output
UPEP	Urine protein electropheresis
UPPP	Uvulopalatopharyngeoplasty
URI	Upper respiratory tract infection
US	Ultrasound
UTD	Up to date
UTI	Urinary tract infection
UV	Ultraviolet

V	Vomiting
VA	Visual acuity
VATS	Video-assisted thoracoscopic surgery
VAX	Vaccine
VBAC	Vaginal birth after cesarean section
VBG	Venous blood gas
VC	Vital capacity; vocal cord
VCUG	Voiding cystourethrogram
VF	Ventricular fibrillation
VIP	Vasoactive intestinal peptide
VP	Ventriculoperitoneal
V&P	Vagotomy and pyloroplasty
VS	Vital signs
VSD	Ventricular septal defect
VSS	Vital signs stable
VT	Ventricular tachycardia
VWF	von Willebrand factor
WBAT	Weight bearing as tolerated
WBC	White blood cells
WDWN	Well developed, well nourished
WNL	Within normal limits
W/O	Without
W/U	Workup
X	Except
XLR	Crossed-leg raise
XRT	Radiation therapy
ZE	Zollinger-Ellison (syndrome)

The Hospital

CCU	Coronary care unit; critical care unit
ICF	Intermediate care facility
ICU	Intensive care unit
ECU	Emergency care unit
EMS	Emergency medical service
ER	Emergency room
OT	Operating theatre/theatre

Clinical History

ABCD	Airway, breathing, circulation, defibrillate in cardiopulmonary resuscitation
ABSYS	Above symptoms
AC/a.c.	*Ante cibum* (before a meal)
Ad lib	*Ad libitum* (as desired)
ADR	Adverse drug reaction
BC, BLCO, CBC	(Complete) blood count
BID/b.i.d.	*Bis in die* (twice a day)
BIPRO	Biochemistry profile
BP	Blood pressure
BUCR	BUN and creatinine
CC	Chief complaint
CPE, CPX	Complete physical examination
CVS	Current vital signs
DM	Diastolic murmur
DNR	Do not resuscitate
DOA	Death on arrival
E/A	Emergency admission
EAU	Emergency admission unit
ESR	Erythrocyte sedimentation rate
FEN	Fluid, electrolytes and nutrition
FH, FAHX	Family history
FHVD	Family history of vascular disease
GERS	Gastroesophageal reflux symptoms
GP	General practitioner
H&P	History and physical examination
HARPPS	Heat, absence of use, redness, pain, pus, swelling
IV/i.v.	Intravenous
LUQ	Left upper quadrant (of abdomen)
M.D.	*Medicinae doctor*
MOUS	Multiple occurrence of unexplained symptoms
NBM	Nil by mouth (nothing by mouth, U.K.)
NPO	*Non para os* (nothing by mouth)
p.c.	*Post cibum* (after meals)
p.r.n.	*Pro re nata* (according to circumstances, may require)
PC	Present complaint
PE, Pex, Px, PHEX	Physical examination
PESS	Problem, etiology, signs, and symptoms
PFH	Positive family history
PH, PHx	Past history
PHI	Past history of illness
PO, P.O.	*Per os* (by mouth, orally)
q.2h	*Quaque secunda hora* (every 2 hours)
q.3h	*Quaque tertia hora* (every 3 hours)

q.d.	*Quaque die* (every day)
q.h.	*Quaque hora* (every hour)
q.i.d.	*Quarter in die* (four times daily)
q.v.	*Quantum vis* (as much as desired)
RBC	Red blood count
RDA	Recommended daily allowance
RLL	Right lower lobe (of lungs)
RS, ROS	Review of symptoms
Rx	Prescribe, prescription drug
S	Signs
S&S, S/S, SS	Signs and symptoms
SC, S/C, SQ	Subcutaneous
Si op. sit,	*Si opus sit* (if necessary)
SM	Systolic murmur
SOAP	Subjective, objective, assessment and plan (used in problem-oriented records)
Sx	Symptoms
t.i.d.	*Ter in die* (three times daily)
TPN	Total parenteral nutrition
TWBC	(Total) white blood count
U&E	Urea and electrolytes
UGIS	Upper gastrointestinal symptoms
URELS	Urine electrolytes
VS, vs	Vital signs
VSA	Vital signs absent
VSOK	Vital signs normal
VSS	Vital signs stable
WRS	Work-related symptoms

Cardiology

3D-US	Three-dimensional ultrasound
ACC	American College of Cardiology
AHA	American Heart Association
AVB	Atrioventricular block
CDI	Color Doppler imaging
CEUS	Contrast-enhanced ultrasound
CTA	CT angiography
CVMR	Cardiovascular magnetic resonance
CW Doppler	Continuous-wave Doppler
DFT	Defibrillation threshold
DICOM	Digital imaging and communications in medicine
DSA	Digital subtraction angiography
DTMS	Dipyridamole-thallium myocardial scintigraphy
EBCT	Electron beam CT

EHJ	*European Heart Journal*
EMPS	Exercise myocardial perfusion scintigraphy
ESC	European Society of Cardiology
ET	Electrophysiological testing
Fr	French (unit of a scale for denoting size of catheters)
GEMRA	Gadolinium-enhanced magnetic resonance angiography
HU	Hounsfield units
IACB/IAB	Intra-aortic counterpulsation balloon pump/intra-aortic balloon
IHD	Ischemic heart disease
IVUS	Intravascular ultrasound
JACC	*Journal of the American College of Cardiology*
LAO	Left anterior oblique projection
LOCM	Low-osmolar contrast medium
MPS	Myocardial perfusion scintigraphy
NASPE	North American Society of Pacing and Electrophysiology
NYHA	New York Heart Association
OCT	Optical coherence tomography
PET	Positron emission tomography
PCR	Paris Course on Revascularization
PCWP	Pulmonary capillary wedge pressure
PFO	Patent foramen ovale
PMV	Percutaneous mitral valvulotomy (or valvuloplasty)
PTCA	Percutaneous transluminal coronary angioplasty
PWD	Pulsed-wave Doppler
QCT	Quantitative CT
QCA	Quantitative coronary angiography
RAO	Right anterior oblique projection
RF	Radiofrequency
ROI	Region of interest
SACT	Sinoatrial conduction time
SCAI	Society for Cardiac Angiography and Interventions
SCINT	Scintigraphy
SESC	Sestamibi scan
SND	Sinus node dysfunction
SNRT	Sinus node recovery time
SPECT	Single photon emission computed tomography
SVT	Supraventricular tachycardia
TCT	Transcatheter therapeutics
VF/VT	Ventricular fibrillation/ventricular tachycardia
VRT	Volume rendering technique

Anatomy of the Heart

AS	Atrial septum
AV	Aortic valve
AVN	Atrioventricular node
CS	Coronary sinus
HB	His bundle
IVC	Inferior vena cava
LA	Left atrium
LAA	Left atrium appendage
LAD	Left anterior descending coronary artery
LBB	Left bundle branch
LCX	Left circumflex artery
LMCA	Left main coronary artery
LV	Left ventricle
LVOT	Left ventricle outflow tract
MV	Mitral valve
PV	Pulmonary valve
RA	Right atrium
RBB	Right bundle branch
RCA	Right coronary artery
RV	Right ventricle
SN	Sinus node
SVC	Superior vena cava
TV	Tricuspid valve
VS	Ventricular septum

Exercises: Common Sentences Containing Abbreviations

This section presents common sentences containing abbreviations that have already been described above.

Sentences:

- A 72-year-old female visited our hospital with a CC of chest pain. She was diagnosed as having a LMCA disease and underwent CABG on an emergent basis.
- The platelet and TWBC exceeded their normal ranges.
- A baseline ECG was obtained, and showed RBBB and AF.
- 2D-echo showed an enlargement of the LA, with a PFO.
- He is actually on ACEI, ASA, and statins. Ten years ago he underwent a primary PTCA.
- Approximately 1% of cardiac cells, including those in SN and AVN, are automatic.

- After been admitted at the ICU with a clinical picture of a severe stroke, the US showed a big thrombus in the LAA.
- LMCA stent implantation is still a highly debated issue. Most cardiac surgeons and cardiologists prefer to do CABG surgery in these patients.
- ASD percutaneous closure is an easy, safe, and cost-effective procedure.
- In patients with AF as the baseline heart rhythm, it is not possible to record the A wave of the MV flow, because there is no LA contraction at all.
- When an ACE inhibitor is administered, glomerular filtration is reduced.
- Some investigators use HU to determine the presence of intraluminal thrombus in a coronary artery, assessed by CT scan. However, IVUS and ANGIO, as well, remain the gold-standard methods.
- The patient had an episode of syncope. A rush HS murmur was heard. The ECG showed LVH and the echo revealed a high-gradient AS.
- CHF secondary to AMI and IHD is the most frequent final consequence of tobacco abuse.
- PFO is a frequent cause of consultation in children with mild-to-moderate degree heart murmurs.
- All patients with ASD and PFO must receive antibiotic prophylaxis before a dental extraction because they are at high risk of suffering BE.
- The main cause of mortality in elderly patients presenting with AMI is VF.
- A 30-year-old patient diagnosed of ASD was carried out to the cath lab to get the defect closed. During the diagnostic part of the procedure we saw that the catheter went from the URPV to the SVC. We made a diagnosis of partial abnormal venous drainage and stopped the procedure.
- Beta blockers induce low heart rate by their effect on the SN.

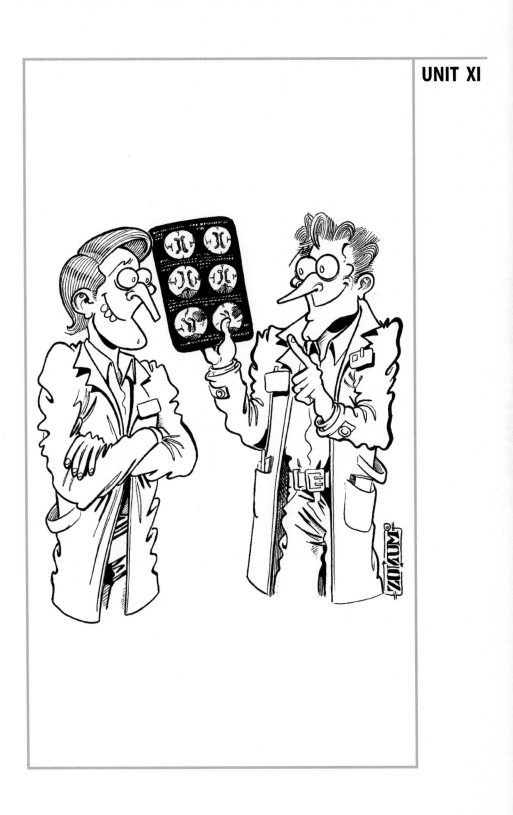

Unit XI Cardiovascular Clinical History

Introduction

Obtaining an accurate history is the first critical step in determining the etiology of a patient's problem. Many times, you will be able to make a diagnosis based on the clinical history alone. The value of the clinical history will depend on your ability to obtain relevant information. Your sense of what constitutes important data has grown exponentially in the past years as you have gained a greater understanding of the pathophysiology of disease through increased exposure to patients and illnesses. However, non-native English-speaking cardiologists may not be in possession of the tools that will enable them to obtain a good clinical history in English. In this chapter, we provide you with some of the basic communication skills we all need to take an appropriate cardiovascular history in English.

Getting Started

Always introduce yourself to the patient.
- Good morning, Mr. Lee. Come and sit down. I'm Dr. Barba.
- Good afternoon, Mrs. Lafontaine. Take a seat, please.

The Chart

Good communication between doctor and patient is vital in order to establish an accurate medical history. Try to make the environment as private and free of distractions as possible. This may be difficult depending on where the interview is taking place. The emergency room and non-private patient rooms are notoriously difficult spots. It would be advisable to find an alternative site for the interview if both these places are noisy and congested. It is also acceptable to politely ask visitors to leave so that you can have some privacy.

In case you were not aware of it, charts are almost entirely written in doctors' shorthand. Get a chart, photocopy it, and go over it thoroughly; the sooner you do it, the better.

If the interview is being conducted in an outpatient setting, then it is probably better to allow the patient to wear his/her own clothing while you chat with them. At the conclusion of the interview, provide the patient with a gown and leave the room while he/she undresses in preparation for the physical exam.

Initial Question(s)

The patient's main physical ailment is usually referred to as the "chief complaint." Perhaps a less pejorative and more accurate nomenclature would be to identify this as their area of "chief concern."

Ideally, you would like to hear patients describe the problem in their own words. Open-ended questions are a good way to get the ball rolling. These include:

• What brings you here?
• How can I help you?
• What seems to be the problem?

Encourage the patients to be as descriptive as possible. While it is simplest to focus on a single, dominant problem, patients occasionally identify more than one issue that they wish to address. When this occurs, explore each one individually using the strategy described below. Some usual forms of invitation to describe symptoms are:

• Well now, what seems to be the problem?
• Well, how can I help you?
• Would you please tell me how I can help you?
• Your GP (general practitioner) says you've been having trouble with your. ... Please tell me about it.
• My colleague Dr. Sanders says your symptoms got worse. Is that correct?

Follow-Up Questions

There is no single best way to question a patient. Successful interviewing requires that you avoid medical terminology and make use of a descriptive language that is familiar to them. There are several broad questions applicable to any complaint:

1. Duration
   a. How long has this condition lasted?
   b. Is it similar to a past problem? If so,
   c. What was done at that time?

2. Severity/character
   a. How bothersome is this problem?
   b. Does it interfere with your daily activities?
   c. Does it keep you up at night?

Invite the patients to rate the problem. If they are describing pain, ask them to rate it from 1 to 10, with 10 being the worse pain of their life (e.g., childbirth, a broken limb, etc.). Ask them to describe the symptom in terms with which they are already familiar. When describing pain, ask if it is like anything else that they have felt in the past. Knife-like? A sensation of pressure? A toothache? If it affects their activity level, then try to determine to what degree this occurs. For example, if they complain of shortness of breath when walking, ask them how many blocks they can walk.

3. Location/Radiation
   a. Is the symptom (e.g., pain) located in a specific place?
   b. Has this changed over time?
   c. If the symptom is not localized, does it spread to other areas of the body?
4. Have they tried any therapeutic maneuvers?
   If so, which ones have made it better (or worse)?

5. Pace of illness
   Is the problem getting better, worse, or staying the same? If it is changing, then what has been the rate of change?

6. Are there any associated symptoms?
   Often times the patient notices other things that have popped up around the same time as the dominant problem.

7. What does the patient think the problem is, and/or what is the patient worried it might be?

8. Why today?
   This is particularly relevant when a patient chooses to make mention of symptoms/complaints that appear to be long standing.
   a. Is there something new/different today as opposed to every other day when this problem has been present?
   b. Does this relate to a gradual worsening of the symptom itself?
   c. Has the patient developed a new perception of its relative importance (e.g., a friend told him/her they should get it checked out)?

The content of subsequent questions will depend on both what you uncover and your understanding of patients and their illnesses. If, for example, the patient's initial complaint was chest pain, then you might have uncovered the following by using the above questions:

The pain began 1 month ago and only occurs with activity. It rapidly goes away with rest. When it does occur, it is a steady pressure focused on the center of the chest that is roughly a 5 (on a scale of 1 to 10). Over the last week, it has happened six times, while in the first week it happened only once. The patient has never experienced anything like this previously and has not mentioned this problem to anyone else prior to meeting with you. No specific therapy has been employed so far.

The Rest of the History

The remainder of the history is obtained after completing the clinical history of present illness (HPI). As such, the previously discussed techniques for facilitating the exchange of information still apply.

Past Medical History

The following questions can help uncover important past events:

- Have you ever received medical care? If so, what problems/issues were addressed?
- Was the care continuous (i.e., provided on a regular basis by a single person) or was it episodic?
- Have you ever undergone any procedures, X-rays, CT scans, MRIs, or other special testing?
- Have you ever been hospitalized? If so, for what?

It is quite amazing how many patients forget what would seem to be important medical events. It is not unusual to find a patient who reports little past history during your interview yet reveals a complex series of illnesses to your resident. These patients are generally not purposefully concealing information. They simply need to be prompted by the right questions!

Past Surgical History

- Have you ever been operated on, even as a child?
- What year did this occur?
- Were there any complications?
- If the patient does not know the name of the operation, then try to determine why it was performed.

Medications

- Do you take any medicines? If so, what is the dose and frequency?
- Do you know why you are being treated?

Medication non-compliance/confusion is a major clinical problem, particularly when regimens are complex, patients older, cognitively impaired, or simply disinterested. It is important to ascertain if they are actually taking the medication as prescribed.

Do not forget to ask about either over the counter or "non-traditional" medications.

- How much are you taking and what are they treating?
- Has it been effective?
- Are these medicines being prescribed by a practitioner? Are they self-administered?

Allergies/Reactions

- Have you ever experienced any adverse reactions to medications?

Smoking History

Have you ever smoked? If so, how many packets per day and for how many years?

If the patient quit:

- When did this occur?

The packets per day multiplied by the number of years gives the pack-years, a widely accepted method for smoking quantification.

Alcohol

- Do you drink alcohol? If so, how much per day and what type of alcohol?

If the patient does not drink on a daily basis, then:

- How much do you consume over a week or month?

Other Drug Use

Any drug use, past or present, should be noted. Get in the habit of asking all your patients these questions, as it can be surprisingly difficult to determine accurately who is at risk strictly based on appearance. Remind them that these questions are not meant to judge but rather to assist you in identifying risk factors for particular illnesses (e.g., HIV, hepatitis). In some cases, however, a patient will clearly indicate that they do not wish to discuss these issues. Respect their right to privacy and move on. Perhaps they will be more forthcoming later.

Obstetric (When Appropriate)

- Have you ever been pregnant? If so, how many times?
- What was the outcome of each pregnancy (e.g., full-term delivery, spontaneous abortion)?

Sexual Activity

This is an uncomfortable line of questioning for many practitioners. However, it can provide important information and should be pursued. As with questions about substance abuse, your ability to determine on sight who is sexually active (and in what type of activity) is rather limited. By asking these questions to all of your patients, the process will become less awkward.

- Do you participate in intercourse?
- Do you participate in sexual intercourse with persons of the same or opposite sex?
- Are you involved in a stable relationship?
- Do you use condoms or other means of birth control?
- Are you married?
- Are you divorced?
- Have you ever suffered from sexually transmitted diseases?
- Do you have children? If so, are they healthy?

Family History

In particular, you are searching for heritable illnesses among first- or second-degree relatives – coronary artery disease, diabetes, and certain malignancies. Patients should be as specific as possible. "Heart disease," for example, includes valvular disorders, coronary artery disease, and congenital abnormalities. Find out the age of onset of the illnesses, as this has prognostic importance for the patient.

Work/Hobbies/Other

- What sort of work do you do, Mr. Lee?
- Have you always done the same thing? Do you enjoy it?
- If retired, what do you do to stay busy? Any hobbies?
- Where are you from originally?

Write-Ups

The written history and physical (H&P) is not an instrument designed to torture medical students and residents. It is an important reference document that gives information to all health providers, and it is an important medicolegal document.

Knowing what to include and what to leave out will be largely dependent on your understanding of illness and of course, of the language you are using. In the United States, then the chart structure follows some guidelines that generally include these items:

- Chief complaint or chief concern (CC)
- History of present illness (HPI)
- Past medical history (PMH)
- Past surgical history (PSH)
- Medications (MEDS)
- Allergies/reactions (All/RXNs)
- Social history (SH)
- Family history (FH)
- Obstetrical history (when appropriate)
- Review of systems (ROS)

The most important ROS questioning (i.e., pertinent positives and negatives related to the chief complaint) is generally noted at the end of the HPI. The responses to a more extensive review that covers all organ systems are placed in this "ROS" area of the write-up. In actual practice, most providers do not document such an inclusive ROS. The ROS questions, however, are the same ones that, in a different setting, are used to unravel the cause of a patient's CC:

- Physical exam
- Lab results, radiological studies, EKG interpretation, etc.
- Assessment and plan

Sample Write-Up

Within this sample, you will find the complete process of evaluation and hospital-admission of a typical cardiologic patient, as usual at university hospitals in the United States.

01/27/07 MEDICAL SERVICE STUDENT ADMISSION NOTE

Location: A-GM

Mr. "S" is a 78 yo man with h/o CHF and CAD, who presented with increasing lower extremity edema and weight gain.

HPI Mr. "S" has a long history of CHF subsequent to multiple MI's last in 2001. Cardiac cath at that time revealed occlusions in LAD, OMB, and circ with EF of 50%. ECHO in 2006 showed a dilated LV, EF of 20–25%, diffuse regional wall motion abnormalities, 2+MR and trace TR. His CHF has been managed medically with captopril, lasix, metolazone, and digoxin. Over the past 6 months, he has required increasing doses of lasix to control his edema. He was seen 2 wks ago by his Cardiologist, at which time he was noted to have leg, scrotal and penile edema. His lasix dose was increased to 120 BID without relief from his swelling.

Over the past week, he and his wife have noticed an increase in his LE edema, which then became markedly worse in the past two days. The swelling was accompanied by a weight gain of 10 lb in 2 days (175 to 185 lb) as well as a decrease in his exercise tolerance. He now becomes dyspneic when rising to get out of bed and has to rest due to SOB when walking on flat ground. He has 2-pillow orthopnea, denies PND. His chronic cough has worsened and is now productive of "transparent" sputum with no hemoptysis. He has audible wheeze. Denies CP/pressure/palpitations/diaphoresis. No nausea/no vomiting. He eats in limited quantities and drinks 6–8 glasses liquid/day. Urinary frequency has increased but the amount urinated has decreased. He states he has been taking all prescribed medications.

PMH

CHF: as above
MI
A-fib: on Coumadin
Pacemaker placed in 3/03 for a-fib/-flutter and slow ventricular response
HTN
Chronic renal insufficiency: BUN/Cr stable on 1/21/04, 52/1.4
DM: controlled with glyburide. Admitted for hypoglycemia in 9/06

PSH
Tonsillectomy
MED
Lasix 120 mg BID
Metolazone 5 mg daily
Captopril 50 mg TID
Digoxin 0.125 mg daily
KCl
Coumadin 4 mg daily
Glyburide 2.5 mg BID
Colace 100 mg BID

All/RXNs
No known drug allergies.

SH
Married for 45 years; sexual active with wife. Three children, 2 grandchildren, all healthy and well; all live within 50 miles. Retired school teacher. Enjoys model car building. Walks around home, shopping but otherwise not physically active.

FH
Sister and mother with DM, father with CAD, age onset 50. Brother with leukemia.

PE (Also see Unit 12, Cardiovascular examination).
VS: T 97.1, P65, BP 116/66, O2 Sat 98% on 2L NC
GEN: elderly man lying in bed with head up, NAD
HEENT: NCAT, multiple telangiectasias on face and nose, EOMi, PERRL, OP-benign
NECK: thyroid not palpable, no LAD, carotid pulse +2 B, no bruits, no JVD
RESP: +dullness to perc at right base, +ant wheezes, +crackles 1/2 way up chest bilat.
COR: RRR, +2/6 holosystolic murmur at apex radiating to axilla, no gallops
ABD: +BS, distended, nontender, no HSM, liver percussed to 9 cm at MCL
PULSES: 2 femoral B, +1 PT/DP B
EXT: +3 edema to lower back, abdomen including genitals, hyperemia over ant., legs bilat, warm, non-tender; non-clubbing, cyanosis
SKIN: 4-cm ulcer on R buttock with central scabbing, non-tender, no discharge
NEURO: AOX3; difficulty remembering events, dates; remainder of exam nonfocal

LABS/DATA
Na 134, Cl 95, Bun 61, Glu 95, K 3.9, CO_2 40.8, CR 1.4, WBC 9.9, PLT 329, HCT 43.9, Alk phos 72, Tot prot 5.6, Alb 2.5 T Bili 0.5, ALT 17, AST 52, LDH 275, CPK 229
CXR: mildly prominent vessels. Minimal interstitial congestion. Cardiomegaly, no infiltrates.

ECHO 1/27:
LV mild dilated (ED = 6 cm) severely depressed global systolic function with EF 20–25%. Extensive area thinning and akinesis: anterior, anteroseptal, anterolateral c/w old infarct
2. Mod 2-3/4 MR. LA size nl
3. No AS/AI
4. RV dilated with preserved fxn. 2-3/4 TR. PA pressure 36+ RA pressure.

ASSESSMENT/PLAN
72-year-old man with h/o CHF following MI, chronic renal insufficiency, and venous stasis admitted with worsening edema and DOE. His symptoms are most consistent with increasing CHF-biventricular, which would account for both his pulmonary congestion as well as his peripheral edema. His renal disease is a less likely explanation for his extensive edema as his BUN/Cr has remained stable throughout. However, his low albumin, which could contribute to his edema, may be due to renal losses.

So if his edema is due to CHF, why has it become gradually and now acutely worse? Possibilities include: 1) worsening LV function, 2) another MI, 3) worsening valvular disease, 4) poor compliance with medications, or 5) excess salt and water intake. His echo today shows no change in his EF, but there is marked wall motion abnormalities with akinesis. There is no evidence in his history, EKG, or enzymes for current ischemia/infarct. He does have MR and TR and his valvular disease may in part account for his worsening symptoms though his estimated PA pressure is unchanged, and his LA is not dilated. The most likely cause of his failure is a combination of poor compliance with medication and fluid overload from excessive intake. We will continue to investigate the possibility of a structural precipitant for his deterioration and treat his current symptoms.

1. Pulm: his wheezing, crackles, and oxygen requirement are all likely due to pulmonary congestion from LV dysfunction. He has no signs, symptoms of pulm infection.
   O_2 to maintain sat greater than 95%.
   Treat cardiac disease as below.
2. Cardiac: As above, his picture is consistent with CHF with no clear precipitant. Will continue to evaluate structural disease as precipitating factor and treat fluid overload.
   Strict I/O's, daily weights
   Fluid restriction to 1.5L
   Low-salt diet
   Lasix 80 mg IV with IV metolatzone now and Q8.. With goal diuresis of 2–3 L/day
   Increase digoxin to 0.25 mg daily
   Continue captopril 50 mg TID
   Check electrolytes, renal function (fxn) and digoxin level in AM
   Education about appropriate diet
   Repeat echo and compare with old film
   Consider Cardiology consult if fails to improve, needs invasive hemodynamic monitoring or cath.
3. GI: Continue Colace
4. Renal: We will continue to evaluate whether he could be losing protein from his kidney leading to his increasing edema. Check urine Prot/Cr ratio.
5. DM: His sugars have been well-controlled on current regimen.
   - Continue glyburide
   - ADA 2,100 calorie diet
   - FS BS ACHS

Signed by:

At the Cardiology Ward

Within the hospital, each branch of medicine has its own structure and approach. Several elements, however, are common to all:

1. Organization. Health care in teaching hospitals is very hierarchical. At the top of the pyramid is the attending physician, a staff doctor who has ultimate responsibility for the patient. Beneath them is the supervising resident, a physician in the advanced stages of their training. Interns, students, visitors, fellows may be also members of the team.
2. Team approach. It is a system of graduated responsibility, allowing less experienced providers the chance to become increasingly involved in the decision making process over time.
3. Role of the student/fellow/resident

   The primary focus of the team is to provide good care for the patient. Within this context, these physicians are also expected to supervise and train others, increase their own knowledge, and provide for your educational needs.

   Work rounds occur each morning and are the time when the team sees each patient, discusses their course, and decides on the diagnostic and therapeutic plan of the day. In order to be maximally efficient, it falls to the students and interns to gather relevant clinical data. This process is referred to as pre-rounding.

Note Writing

The format for the complete H&P is discussed above. Daily notes should be organized so that they are brief, yet highlight important data and clearly express clinical impressions. This, of course, must be done within the context of your knowledge base. As with many of the other tasks in which students participate, notes serve two purposes: They are an actual descriptive document that chronicles the patient's course, and they are a learning tool that allows you to think about what is going on and express organized thoughts. A few things to remember:

- The data presented should be factual.
- The impression and plan generally reflects the thoughts of the entire team.
- The length of the note will depend largely on your experience, understanding of the case and the complexity of the patient's illness.
- Certain services have very particular styles, emphasizing aspects that are important to the care that they provide. Cardiology teams, for example, tend to highlight fluid status, urine output, vital signs and enzymes values. However, to our knowledge, no one has shown that the length of the note correlates with the quality of care delivered.

The basic format is referred to as a "SOAP note." This stands for the major categories included within the note: *s*ubjective information, *o*bjective data, *a*ssessment, and *p*lan.

A sample note for a patient receiving treatment for pneumonia after a CABG is as follows:

Hospital day #12

S: Patient feeling less short of breath, with decreased cough and sputum production. Mild sternum pain.

O: Maximum Temperature: 101.5 (yesterday 103)
- Pulse: 80–90
- BP: 110–120/70–80, RR: 20–24 Sat: 95% 2L O_2 (yesterday 95% 4L O_2)
- I/O: 2.5 L IV, 1 L PO/UO 2L, BM × 1 Wt 140 lbs (no change from yesterday)

Day #3 ceftriaxone, 1 g IV BID

PE: No JVD
Lungs: Crackles and dullness to percussion at R base with egophony; no change c/w yesterday
C/V: S_1 S_2, no S_3, S_4, m
Abd: soft, non-tender
Ext: no edema
Labs: Sputum and blood Cx still negative; otherwise, no new data

Assessment/Plan:
- Post-operative RLL Pneumonia: Responding to IV ceftriaxone, with decreasing O_2 requirement and fever curve. Also feeling better. No evidence of complications.
  Plan:
  - IV Abx × 1 addl day ... then change to PO Azithromax
  - Hep. lock IV to assess if PO intake adequate
  - Check sat off O_2 ... d/c if under 92%
  - Encourage ambulation
  - Consider discharge in approximately 2 days if continues to improve

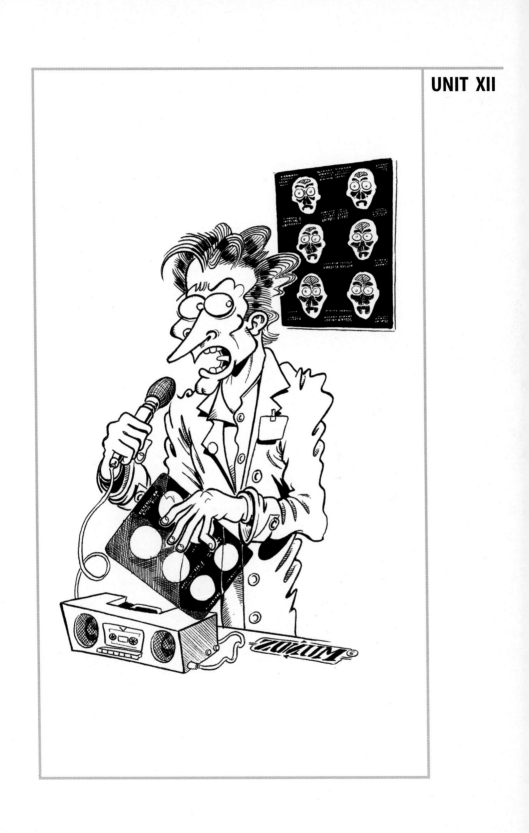

Unit XII   Cardiovascular Examination

Patient Examination

Instructions for Undressing

- Would you slip off your top things, please?
- Slip off your coat, please.
- Would you mind taking off all your clothes except your underwear? (Men)
- Please would you take off all your clothes except your underwear and bra? (Women)
- You should take off your underwear, too.
- Lie on the couch and cover yourself with the blanket.
- Lie on the stretcher with your shoes and socks off, please.
- Roll your sleeve up, please; I'm going to take your blood pressure.

Instructions for Position on Examining Table

- Make yourself comfortable on the table and lie on your back (supine position).
- Lie down please (supine position).
- Roll over onto your tummy (from supine to prone position).
- Lie on your tummy please (prone position)
- Please turn over and lie on your back again.
- Bend your left knee.
- Straighten your leg again.
- Roll over onto your left side.
- Sit with your legs dangling over the edge of the couch.
- Lie down with your legs stretched in front of you.
- Sit up and bend your knees.
- Lean forward.
- Get off the table ("Get off" is sometimes perceived as too informal and impolite).
- Please come off the table.

- Please sit up.
- Get off the table and stand up.
- Stand up from the table.
- Stand up please.
- Lie on your back.
- Lie on your tummy and relax.
- Let yourself go loose.

Questions and Commands

- Open your mouth please.
- Raise your arm.
- Raise it more.
- Say it once again.
- Stick out your tongue.
- Swallow please.
- Take a deep breath.
- Take a deep breath and hold it in.
- Breath normally.
- Grasp my hand.
- Try again.
- Bear down as if for a bowel movement (Valsalva maneuver).
- Please lie on your tummy (prone position).
- Walk across the room.

Instructions to Get Dressed

- You can get dressed now. Take your time; we are not in a hurry.
- Please get dressed. Take your time; we are not in a hurry.

Cardiovascular Examination

- Level of consciousness
  - Altered level of consciousness
  - GCS (Glasgow Coma Scale)
  - Loss of consciousness
  - Alert and oriented

- Vital signs
  - Heart rate
  - Blood pressure
  - Respiratory frequency
  - Oxygen saturation

- Circulation
  - Carotid pulses, quality and symmetry. Murmurs
  - Jugular pulse ("a" and "w" waves)
  - Thrills, lifts, and waveforms
  - Heart sounds (first and second sound characteristics are always described; third and fourth – summation gallop – are described when present)
    - Normal
    - Intensity
    - Dampening
    - Loudness
      - Accentuated
      - Decreased intensity
    - Split
      - Wide splitting of the first heart sound
      - Persistent splitting of second heart sound
      - Paradoxical splitting of second heart sound
    - Ejection sounds (clicks)
      - Pulmonary ejection sound
      - Aortic ejection sound
    - Non-ejection systolic sound
      - Mid-systolic clicks are part of the spectrum of the mitral valve prolapse syndrome.
    - Opening snaps
      - Opening snap of mitral valve stenosis
    - Presystolic impulse
    - Pericardial knock (early diastolic sound of constrictive pericarditis)
    - Pericardial friction rub
    - Cardiovascular murmurs
      - Systolic
      - Diastolic
      - Continuous
      - Musical
      - Low- or high-pitched
      - Blowing
      - Harsh
      - Rumbling (diastolic rumble of MS)
      - Honking
  - Bedside maneuvers
    - Respiration
    - Isometric exercise (handgrip)
    - Valsalva maneuver
- Breathing
  - Rhythm
  - Depth
  - Adequate

- Shallow
- Deep
- Quality
- Easy
- Labored
- Stridor
- Painful
- Dyspnea
- Rales
- Rhonchi
- Sibilants
- Pleural rub
- Liver and spleen enlargement
- Peripheral pulses
- Ascites
- Ankle edema

No Treatment

- There is nothing wrong with you. (It may be a quirk of the US health-care system, but we are encouraged to validate a patient's complaints. Hence, even if nothing objective is identified, the patient's symptoms are still acknowledged. For example, I might say, "I understand that you have chest pain. The 2D echo and stress test does not show any abnormality or anything that requires treatment. Our next step will be to. ...")
- This will clear up on its own.
- This illness is self-limited and will resolve on its own.
- There doesn't seem to be anything wrong with your heart.

Typical Sentences Regarding Heart-Auscultation Findings

- Corrigan first reported the early diastolic sound of constrictive pericarditis, the so-called pericardial knock.
- The opening snap of the mitral valve may be difficult to differentiate from other sounds.
- Third and fourth sounds often are intermittent and may be accentuated by exercise.
- In patients with aortic and mitral valve prostheses, the development of severe incompetence of the aortic valve prosthesis may alter the intensity of the closing sound of the mitral valve prosthesis.
- Disk valves produce clear, crisp, closing sounds.
- A brief mid-systolic crescendo–decrescendo murmur is audible.

- Auscultation should begin at the right second parasternal interspace, with the diaphragm.
- The murmurs and heart sounds generated in the left side of the heart decrease on inspiration and are best heard during expiration.
- The first heart sound in patients with secundum atrial septal defect is normal.
- Regarding pulmonary stenosis, the more severe the stenosis, the more widely split the second sound will be.
- The murmur of tricuspid insufficiency is heard best over the xyphoid or along the fourth and fifth left parasternal areas.
- A diastolic murmur of low to medium frequency occasionally is heard in patients with idiopathic pulmonary artery dilatation.
- A late systolic murmur, either isolated of accompanied by a non-ejection click, is now considered the classic finding of mitral valve prolapse.
- Thrills rarely accompany aortic diastolic murmurs but may occur in patients with aortic cusp rupture or aortic dissection.
- When the murmur is musical, low in frequency, or has a "seagull sound," then other causes of aortic regurgitation should be considered.
- The rub is best described as a superficial, scratchy, rough sound, occasionally with a coarse, leathery quality, which is heard well when the patient is holding his breath.
- Paradoxical splitting of the second heart sound may be observed during episodes of ischemic cardiac pain.
- The timing of the click and murmur in systole is influenced by left ventricular volume during systole.
- A decrescendo diastolic murmur heard best along the left sternal border is considered to be due to pulmonary valve incompetence.
- The aortic component of the second heart sound may be normal in mild aortic stenosis.
- The murmur of aortic valve stenosis begins after the first sound or after the ejection sound if one is present.

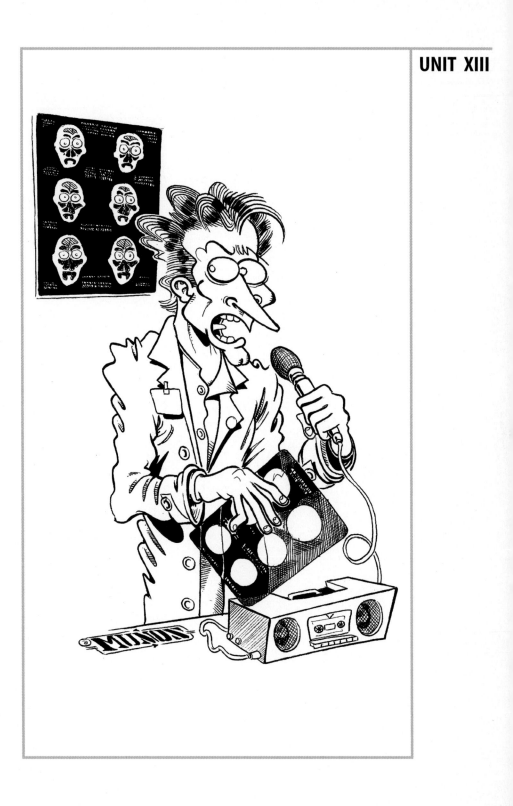

Unit XIII   Prescribing Medication

Introduction

Specifying the therapeutic objective allows physicians to direct prescribing to a clear goal with expected outcomes. For a non–native English-speaking doctor, it is a challenge and a task of utmost medical responsibility to inform clearly about the effect, secondary effects, treatment duration, and dosage to patients.

The World Health Organization (WHO) guide suggests that physicians develop a formulary of personal drugs (P-drugs). P-drugs are effective, inexpensive, well-tolerated drugs that physicians regularly prescribe to treat common problems. Every foreign cardiology resident should have a formulary of P-drugs.

The National Coordinating Council on Medication Error Reporting and Prevention recommends the elimination of most abbreviations for medication instructions, such as QD (daily), QID (four times daily), and QOD (every other day), and drug names such as MSO_4 (morphine sulfate). To be effective, prescribers should eliminate non-standard abbreviations that are easily misread, such as non-English characters (e.g., μ). Using plain English for all prescription writing allows the patient to read and draw attention to any errors.

Most patients at the cardiologist office need not only medication, but also a lot of instructions regarding lifestyle such as giving-up smoking, dietary habits, physical exercise, etc. Non–native English prescribers must be fluent in order to reassure the patient and his/her family regarding complete treatment.

Talking to the Patient about Medication

Talking to Older Patients

Persons age 65 and older account for less than 15% of the US population but consume about a third of all retail prescriptions. They also purchase at least 40% of all non-prescription medicines. When you see older patients, chances are that they have been prescribed medicines by other physicians and take several non-prescription drugs. They may also be more sensitive to effects of medications and may not be able to tolerate adult dosages.

Better communication with these patients can decrease their risks and produce better outcomes. Use these tips when talking to older patients:

- Involve them in choosing and following their medication regimen.
- Review proper dosing schedules with patients and their caregivers.
- If a device is involved, let both the patient and caregiver use it before you several times.
- Ask patients about their medicines each time you see them.
- Ask about medicines prescribed by other physicians.
- Ask about non-prescription medicines.
- Ask about vitamins and nutritional supplements.
- Mention common side effects and ask patients about their experiences.
- Conduct medication checkups with older patients involving all of their medications, prescription, and OTC (over the counter), at least once a year. Provide written instructions when possible.
- Explain the importance of lifestyle changes in addition to medication.
- Ask patients each time you see them if they have any questions or concerns they would like to discuss.
- Speak plainly and make sure they understand by having them repeat instructions.

Counseling a Patient about Drug Therapy

- Always stress the critical nature of adherence to health outcomes. If your patient is adherence-challenged, talk about pillboxes, bottle reminders, and even pager-based systems to make sure that your patient will take the medicines.
- Briefly explain the nature of the disorder and its treatment. Use language the average person can understand.
- Provide educational material about the disorder. If the disorder is chronic (diabetes, hypertension), then explain the need to continue drug therapy indefinitely, possibly for life.
- Briefly explain the name and nature of the drug(s) you are prescribing. Stress the importance of strictly following the instructions for the medicine. Tell the patient about potential adverse effects.
- Explain the need for follow-up visits to monitor the effects of drug treatment and the course of the disorder.
- Explain that drugs may not work in practice exactly as expected. Tell the patient to be alert to the possibility that a new symptom or sign may be drug-related. If one of your patients does have a novel adverse drug reaction, it is critical that you call the US Food and Drug Administration (FDA) MedWatch at 1-800-332-1088 (provided you be in the United States).

- Encourage the patient to call if he/she should feel the need to do so about any aspect of drug treatment. Adjust drug selection and/or dosage regimens to fit individual patients.
- Give special attention to older patients on drug therapy. The elderly generally use multiple drugs concurrently and are more likely to have adverse drug effects.
- If you refer any of your patients to another physician, be certain to obtain a repeat medication history when they return to your care. Check for duplications in medicines by cross-referencing brand or generic names.

Example:

Mr. Ohtonen, you have a stent implanted on your LAD. As you know, it is a DES (drug-eluting stent), and to avoid thrombotic complications you need to be on a combined antiplatelet regime for, at least, 6 months. Clopidogrel, 75 mg one pill daily at lunchtime, along with ASA 100 mg, one pill daily at lunchtime. Besides this, we need to control your blood pressure, so we'll continue on enalapril 5 mg and bisoprolol 2.5 mg, as before the admission. Remember that bisoprolol has some secondary effects that you have already noticed (fatigue and sexual dysfunction). Should you have any other problems, please contact me as soon as you can. Here you have your complete written prescription with my phone number at the bottom.

Patients like Mr. Ohtonen with diabetes and the added diagnosis of hypertension should be informed that enalapril will reduce his blood pressure, protect his kidneys, and could cause a rare but serious reaction called angioedema, which demands immediate medical attention. He should also know that approximately 1 in 15 patients experiences cough, with or without altered taste sensation. When communicating risk, you must use absolute numbers (e.g., 1 in 15), rather than percentages, probabilities, odds, or likelihoods.

Nonpharmacologic therapy remains an important treatment option. Patients with diabetes and the added diagnosis of hypertension may not need medication if they lose weight and exercise.

Prescribing Medication Safely

Although for the beginner, using abbreviations may give a piece of self-esteem and confidence, experts recommend to avoid prescribing with abbreviations, not only at your office, but at the hospital wards too. Some nurses' and pharmacologists' associations have developed prescription guidelines that recommend not to obey a medical order if it includes abbreviations. Here we enunciate some of the most modern recommendations in the field of safely prescribing:

Must Use	Never Use the Following
No zero after a whole number (e.g., 2 mg)	Trailing zero after a whole number (e.g., 2.0 mg)
Zero for all numbers less than one (e.g., 0.2 mg)	Decimal point without a leading zero (e.g., 2 mg)
Metric system (mg, grams, or g, etc.)	Apothecary symbols (drams, grains, etc.)
Units (written out)	U
Micrograms (written out)	Mcg or μg
Hours (h, hr, hrs)	Degree sign (°) for hours
Minutes (min), seconds (sec)	Apostrophe for time (e.g., ' or ")
Twice a week (designate days of week)	BIW
Three times a week (designate days of week)	TIW
Every other day	QOD
At	@

Minimum Standard for Medication Order

Physicians/licensed independent practitioners are responsible to write clear, legible orders. All medication orders must contain the following components to meet the required minimum standard:

- Legible handwriting. Consider printing the order.
- Patient name, medical record number, unit (patient location)
- Date and time (military time)
- A legible signature and identification number for a physician/licensed independent practitioner
- Drug name (written out completely)
- Dosage
- Route
- Frequency or rate (include parameters for PRN)
- Weight in those orders where necessary (antimicrobial form, pediatric patients)

Orders for Nursing Units

Verbal orders – those spoken aloud in person or by telephone – offer more room for error than orders that are written or sent electronically. Once received, a verbal order must be transcribed as a written order, which adds complexity and risk to the ordering process. Some organizations have compiled reports of medical errors caused by verbal orders. A review of these reports indicates that when a nurse relays a verbal order to the pharmacist, the risk of error is even greater. The pharmacist must rely on the accuracy of the nurse's written transcription of the order and the nurse's pronunciation of the drug's name.

Issues that affect the accuracy of verbal orders and contribute to medical errors include the following:

- Sound-alike drug names. There have been numerous reports submitted to control units at US hospitals in which drug names were misheard, resulting in administration of the wrong medications. For example, in one instance a misheard verbal order led to a patient receiving Klonopin (a brand-name for clonazepam, an anticonvulsant) instead of clonidine (an antihypertensive).
- Misinterpreted numbers. In one reported case, an emergency room nurse thought that a physician had stated a patient was to receive "1 and 1/2 teaspoons" of Zithromax, which was given. The written order indicated the dose was 1/2 teaspoon. In a similar case reported to the Institute for Safe Medication Practices (ISMP), an ER physician verbally ordered "hydralazine 15 mg IV," but the nurse heard "hydralazine 50 mg IV," and the patient shocked.
- Verbal communication of multiple medications at the same time. While awaiting transfer of a premature baby girl to a nearby children's hospital, a physician gave a verbal order to administer ampicillin 200 mg and gentamicin 5 mg IV push. According to the same issue of Medication Safety Alert!, the nurse misheard the second antibiotic order as gentamicin 500 mg.

Safe Practices

The following are some safe practices that might be feasible for any hospital:

- Limit verbal communication of prescription or medication orders to urgent situations in which immediate written or electronic communication is not feasible.
- Write down the complete order or enter it into a computer, read it back, and receive confirmation from the person who gave the order.
- Include the purpose of the drug in all medication orders to ensure that the order makes sense in the context of the patient's condition.
- Include the mg/kg dose and the patient's specific dose for all verbal neonatal/pediatric medication orders.
- Ensure that medication doses are expressed in units of weight (mg, g, mEq, mmol).
- Have a second person listen to a verbal order whenever possible.
- Record verbal orders directly onto an order sheet in the patient's chart.

- Disallow verbal requests for medications from nursing units to the pharmacy, unless the verbal order has been transcribed onto an order form and simultaneously faxed or otherwise seen by a pharmacist before medication is dispensed.
- Limit verbal orders to formulary drugs.

Emergency, Do-Not-Resuscitate Orders

A do-not-resuscitate (DNR) order tells medical professionals not to perform CPR. This means that doctors, nurses, and emergency medical personnel will not attempt emergency CPR if the patient's breathing or heartbeat stops. A DNR order is only a decision about CPR and does not relate to any other treatment.

Otherwise, if a DNR has not been signed and a "Code Blue" comes in, the medical team is obliged to start a CPR.

The following phrases are some colloquial words used in such a serious condition as a heartbeat stop. As a cardiologist or a cardiology resident, you already have experienced the feelings and emotional stress linked to the fact that the patient, to whom you said "good morning" a few hours ago, is now leaving this world while your team of doctors, nurses, and students is trying to bring him back.

- Code Blue, room 312!!! Code Blue, room 312!!! Code Blue, room 312!!!
- Alright folks, let's roll him over and put him on the monitor, please!
- You!! Get an ambu bag and start bagging!
- You!! Load me up an 8.0 ET tube and get me the 4.0 MAC and the biggest McGill blade we have, just in case.
- You, grab the crash cart!
- Quick look paddle! "He's in fib!" "Let's juice him!"
- Charging up to 200! "Everybody clear!"
- "Keep the paddles on, please."
- "OK, idioventricular. No carotid pulse. You feel anything down there?" (to another one who was checking for a femoral pulse)
- "Start CPR! " Tube him."
- "Give 1 amp of bicarb."
- "And push 1 of epi and 1 of atropine!"
- "Give 300 of amiodarone, too!"
- "Somebody grab me his chart, read out all of his allergies, meds on the MAR, and his latest labs!"
- "Get me a central line or a Quentin cath!"
- "ROSC! (Pronounced "rosky," for return of spontaneous circulation). He's got a pulse!"
- "Check for a BP, and get me an EKG. Someone call for a portable chest (X-ray), please. Lidocaine drip, too."

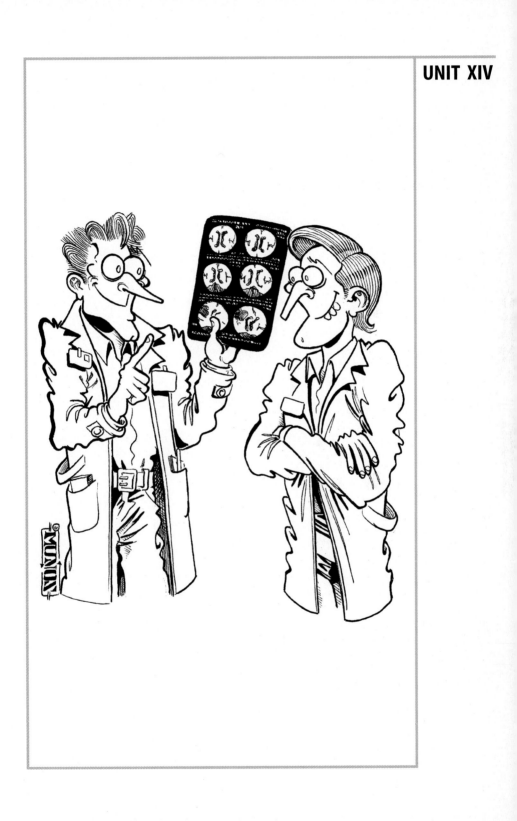

Unit XIV   Echocardiography

Introduction

Although ultrasound medical English shares with multidetector CT, Cardiac magnetic resonance, and cardiac nuclear medicine, many anatomical and pathophysiological terms, the terminology regarding technical aspects of each imaging modality is so different that an ultrasonographer can find difficult to understand the technical nuances of a talk on MDCT, CMR, or cardiac nuclear medicine, even in his/her own native tongue. The concept of "pitch," for example, is something as simple for a cardiologist doing CT as the term "double inversion recovery" for a cardiologist doing MR, but it is likely that many cardiologists who are not doing either multislice CT or cardiac MR are not familiar with these terms.

CT, MR, and nuclear medicine terminology is out of the scope of this manual, and we focus on echocardiography because it is precisely in this real-time, non-invasive imaging modality where the cardiologists must communicate directly with patients.

CT and MR terminology is extensively covered in the book *Radiological English* (R. Ribes, P. Ros, 2007, Springer Publishing, ISBN: 3540293280).

Talking to the Patient

Let us remember some key sentences which will help you to communicate with the patient before, during and after the procedure.

- Would you mind taking off your shirt? (Men)
- Would you please take off your shirt and bra? (Women)
- Please lie on the exam table and roll over onto your left side.
- This is a little bit cold (probe and gel), but it will not harm you.
- Hold your breath please.
- Lie on your back again please.
- Take a deep breath and hold it please.
- Breathe normally.
- Stand up please

- You can get dressed now. Take your time; we are not in a hurry.
- Please get dressed. Take your time.

Transesophageal echocardiography needs more information and patient reassurance. Some additional sentences and commands are:

- With this spray, I will spread your pharynx with local anesthetic. You will feel better and will not have nausea or vomiting.
- Open your mouth please.
- Sting your tongue please.
- Try to swallow the probe. It is easy. It will not harm you.
- Let the saliva drop out. Do not try to swallow now. Breathe normally through your mouth.

Standard Reports

According to the American Society of Echocardiography, the adult transthoracic echocardiography report should be comprised of the following sections:

1. Demographic and other identifying information
   a. Patient's name
   b. Age
   c. Gender
   d. Indications for test
   e. Height
   f. Weight
   g. Referring physician identification
   h. Interpreting physician identification
   i. Date on which the study is performed
   j. Echo study media location (e.g., disk or tape number, etc.)
   k. Date on which the study was ordered, read, transcribed and verified
   l. Location of the patient (inpatient, outpatient, etc.)
   m. Location where the study was performed
   n. Name or identifying information for persons performing the study (e.g., sonographer, physician)
   o. Echo instrument identification
   p. Imaging views obtained, or not obtained (especially if the study is suboptimal)

2. Echocardiographic (Doppler, if indicated) evaluation
   a. Cardiac structures: The following cardiac and vascular structures are evaluated as part of a comprehensive adult transthoracic echocardiography report:

    i. Left ventricle
   ii. Left atrium
  iii. Right atrium
   iv. Right ventricle
    v. Aortic valve
   vi. Mitral valve
  vii. Tricuspid valve
 viii. Pulmonic valve
   ix. Pericardium
    x. Aorta
   xi. Pulmonary artery
  xii. Inferior vena cava and pulmonary veins

b. Measurements: Generally, quantitative measurements are preferable. However, it is recognized that qualitative or semi-quantitative assessments are often performed and frequently adequate. The following types of measurements are commonly included in a comprehensive echocardiography report:
   i. Left ventricle:
      1. Size: dimensions or volumes, at end-systole and end-diastole
      2. Wall thickness and/or mass: ventricular septum and left ventricular posterior wall thicknesses (at end-systole and end-diastole) and/or mass (at end-diastole)
      3. Function: assessment of systolic function and regional wall motion. Assessment of diastolic function
   ii. left atrium:
      1. Size: area or dimension
  iii. Aortic root:
      1. Dimension
   iv. Valvular stenosis:
      1. For valvular stenosis: assessment of severity. Measurements that provide an accurate assessment of severity include trans-valvular gradient and area.
      2. For subvalvular stenosis: Assessment of severity. Measurement of subvalvular gradient provides the most accurate assessment of severity and is therefore recommended.
    v. Valvular regurgitation: Assessment of severity with semi-quantitative descriptive statements and/or quantitative measurements
   vi. Prosthetic valves:
      1. Transvalvular gradient and effective orifice area
      2. Description of regurgitation, if present.
  vii. Cardiac shunts: assessment of severity. Measurements of Qp/Qs (pulmonary-to-systemic flow ratio) and/or orifice area or diameter of the defect are often helpful.

c. Descriptive statements: These descriptive statements are broad in scope, but not all-inclusive, and are provided as an illustrative guide.

Since these statements represent the universe of possible findings, they are not intended to be included in any single report. Rather, a carefully selected subset of these statements should be included in each report, balancing the needs for conciseness and completeness in responding to the patient's and referring physician's needs.

3. Summary: A summary of the echocardiographic report often includes statements that:
   a. Answer the question(s) posed by the referring physician
   b. Emphasize abnormal findings
   c. Compare important differences and similarities of the current study versus previous echocardiographic studies, or reports, if available

Teaching Residents

- This four-chamber view shows a heavily calcified mitral annulus.
- LV ejection fraction is within normal limits.
- We cannot measure the PA systolic pressure. There is no tricuspid regurgitation.
- Please obtain a clearer sub-xyphoid view so we can see the septum.
- The left-ventricle filling pattern is typical of abnormal relaxation.
- Please widen (shorten) the color-ROI.
- The sample volume is not in a proper position. Locate it 1 cm over the mitral plane.
- That rounded image in the apex of the LV could be an old thrombus.
- The anterior wall is clearly akinetic. The other segments contract normally.
- The suprahepatic veins flow is inverted. This suggests a severe tricuspid regurgitation (TR) is present.
- That augmented velocity at that level suggests the presence of an aortic coarctation.
- The mitral regurgitation is severe according to this PISA value.
- There is a mild pericardial effusion without tamponade signs.
- For this baby boy, I prefer to use a 7S probe instead of the 3S.
- The aliasing in the pulmonary artery is typical of a PDA.

Stress Test

There is a wide variety of stress tests described heretofore, which has been employed and evaluated in order to assess myocardial function and to diagnose ischemic heart disease. Since the Master's test at the very beginning, up to the transesophageal electrical stimulation of the right atrium, including dobutamine infusion, adenosine infusion, mental stress, etc.

However, the most accepted and employed method nowadays is the exercise stress test using a treadmill or a bicycle. Sometimes, we make "stress-echo," which combines the treadmill or bicycle part with a rapid capture of echocardiographic images at the end of exercise.

Talking to the Patient

- Good morning Mr. Lewis. We are going to do a stress test. This is a simple test and will not harm you at all. We need you to walk on this treadmill, which will increase its slope and velocity in a stepwise manner, controlled by me. The nurse here, Sandra, will take your blood pressure every 3 minutes. We will be looking at your EKG recording all the time. Should you feel any chest pain, shortness of breath, dizziness, etc., please let me know. We can stop anytime if needed.
- Would you please sign this form? It is the informed consent sheet. Take your time to read it. I can answer to your questions and solve your doubts.
- Please grab this bar gently just to keep your stability. Relax your shoulders. Keep on walking. There is no need to run.
- Are you OK? Any discomfort? Any chest pain?
- Well, that's it. Please slow down. Breathe deeply.

Standard Reports

The stress-test report should be comprised of the following sections:
- Demographic and other identifying information
    - Patient's name
    - Age
    - Gender
    - Indications for test
    - Height
    - Weight
    - Referring physician identification
    - Interpreting physician identification
    - Detailed medication taken by the patient
    - Date of the procedure
- Test data
    - Rest EKG description
    - Protocol (Bruce, etc.)
    - Effort duration (time)
    - Basal and peak heart rate reached and percentage of the theoretical maximum heart rate
    - Basal and peak blood pressure (mmHg)
    - Work load (METS)

- Reason to stop (maximum heart rate, chest pain, dizziness, lack of co-operation, etc.)
- EKG findings (ST-segment behavior, arrhythmias, etc.)
- Summary and conclusions

Head-Up Tilt Test

This is a test used to determine the cause of fainting spells (syncope). The test involves being tilted, always with the head-up, at different angles for a period. Heart rhythm, blood pressure, and other symptoms are closely monitored and evaluated with changes in position.

Talking to the Patient

- Mrs. Robinson, during the test you will lay on a special bed that has a footboard and a motor, which we control so that it can tilt to different degrees.
- The nurse will start an intravenous line in your arm to give you medications and fluids during the procedure, if necessary to treat your symptoms and/or blood pressure and heart rate changes.
- The nurse will connect you to several monitors for monitoring your EKG, blood pressure, respiration, and blood oxygen saturation.
- You will be awake but will be asked to lie quietly and keep your legs still.
- It is important to report your symptoms as they occur. You may feel no symptoms at all; but may feel symptoms of lightheadedness, nausea, dizziness, palpitation, or blurred vision; or you may faint.
- We will give you a medication called X. This medication may make you feel nervous, jittery, or that your heart is beating faster or stronger.
- This feeling will go away as the medication wears off. Your blood pressure, heart rate, and symptoms will be closely monitored and evaluated.

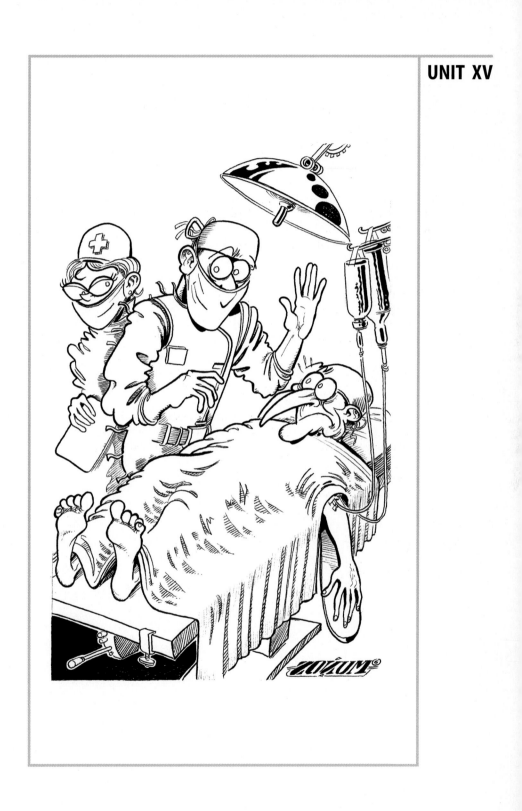

Unit XV   Invasive Cardiac Imaging: the Cath Lab

Introduction

Cath labs (interventional cardiology [IC] suites) are real-time, decision-making environments in which lack of fluency can be troublesome not only for the non–native English-speaking cardiologist, but also for anybody else in the laboratory, the patient included. This is the reason why we have dedicated a complete unit to interventional cardiology.

When you enter an IC suite, your listening skills are much more important than are your fluency; nobody is expecting you to say too much, but everybody takes for granted that you understand them, and that is not always true. You will find no difficulty when the conversation is on the pathology itself; in the first few days many jargon terms, acronyms, and abbreviations can be tricky but with a bit of help, you will soon feel reasonably confident.

If you have not worked in an American hospital, you probably do not know what a SOAP note is. SOAP stands for *s*ubjective comments on the patient, *o*bjective findings, *a*ssessment, and *p*lan, and SOAP note refers to the standard follow-up chart entries. Moreover, many procedures are done nowadays at the cath lab by interventional cardiologists, electrophysiologists, and vascular surgeons. Primary coronary angioplasty, in the myocardial infarction scenario is an emergency that gives no time to language inaccuracies, and it has become the keystone of interventional cardiology practice around the world. But "coronary angiography" language is needed only by interventionalists. Percutaneous valvulotomy, closure devices for atrial and ventricular septal defects, treatment of patent ductus arteriosus, and septal embolization for hypertrophic cardiomyopathy are among the armamentarium of interventional cardiologists.

Study and treatment of arrhythmias using catheters and ablators, implantation of electrical devices as pacemakers and defibrillators, need other language skills completely different from those used by interventional cardiologists performing angioplasty and stenting.

One of the main problems of non–native English-speaking interventional cardiologists working in English-speaking cath labs is the lack of knowledge of basic vocabulary, jargon terminology, acronyms, abbreviations, and set phrases.

Let us begin with this simple conversation that may have happened hundreds of times in cath labs. Familiarity with conversations such as the following will help in our first days in an English-speaking IC suite:

- Cardiologist getting ready for case, speaking to a nurse: "I'll be in as soon as I get the cap, facemask, and booties on."
- Nurse: "I'll have your gown ready for you. What size gloves do you take?"
- Cardiologist: "I usually take 8's but I'm going to double-glove for this case, so I'll take 8 under and 8½ on top. Thanks."

The first thing a foreigner notices in an IC suite is that he/she is not familiar with terminology regarding garments since he/she has not asked for garments in English before and because virtually nothing has been written no booties, masks, caps, gowns, etc.

In the following pages, we go over several sentences typical of an IC suite. Those who have not worked in a cath lab abroad and are not going to do so in the future may not see the point in reviewing so many easy set phrases; these sentences are indeed quite easy to understand for an interventional cardiologist independently of his/her English level.

Our advice is to try to read them aloud. By doing this not-that-simple exercise, you will immediately notice that you may not be confident in reading aloud and pronouncing correctly some of the sentences you used to despise as simple. The best way to become familiar with the listening, pronunciation and spelling of these sentences is to write them down and read them aloud.

When during your first days in a foreign cath lab, you hear some of these sentences uttered by native speakers, you will realize how important it was to have heard the sentences before, and you should already have practiced the first sentences you have to say yourself.

Garments

Tools and devices are usually well known by foreign cardiologists since they have read about them in the literature. Garments are a different issue. Since garment terminology is so engrained in the core of the subspecialty, it is quite difficult to find written garment names; no article is going to say a word on scrubs, booties, masks, lead aprons, radiation badges ...

The most common formula to ask for anything in this environment is:

- Can I have ...?

Everyone who has rotated in an English-speaking cath lab has felt the need to ask for garments:

- Where are the lead aprons?
- Do we have lead aprons?
- This lead apron is too small. Can I have a larger one?
- Can I have a facemask?
- Could you give me a hood?
- Can you let me know where the shoe covers are?
- I'll need a pair of lead gloves.
- What size gloves do you take? 8.
- I'm going to double-glove for this case.
- I'll take 8 under and 8½ on top.
- My scrubs top is soaked. I need to change it.
- There is a blood strain on my scrub pants (British English: trousers).
- I left my radiation badge in my locker.

Look at the schematic representation on the following page in which we have included some of the most common cath lab garments.

Tools and Devices

Once you are properly dressed, you will have to ask for tools and devices. Since most tools and devices are known beforehand, we give you a few examples of usual requests and common formulas to ask for guides, stents, catheters, etc.:

- Can I have a 0.014 guidewire?
- Can I have a hydrophilic guidewire?
- Can I have a 5F introducer?
- Can I have a 16-ga needle?
- Give me a JL4 please.
- Give me a 3×20 balloon please.
- I'd rather use a Swan-Ganz catheter.
- I can now see the stent. I'll use an Amplatz goose neck snare.
- Can I have a torque device?
- Can I have a stiffer guidewire, please?
- Give me the ventricular lead please.
- Let's connect the generator. Double-check the electric threshold.

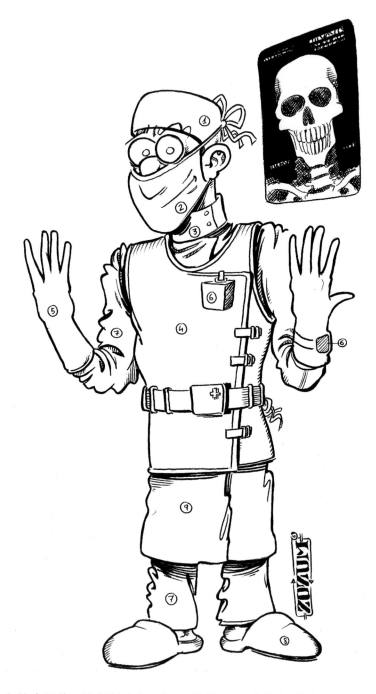

1. Cap, 2. Mask, 3. Thyroid shield, 4. Lead Apron, 5. Gloves, 6. Radiation badge, 7. Scrubs, 8. Clogs, 9. Gown

Talking to the Patient

"Don't breathe, don't move" is probably the commonest command in an IC suite.

- Keep still.
- Don't breathe, don't move.
- Push as if you were going to have a bowel movement (Valsalva maneuver).
- Take a deep breath and hold your breath.
- Let me know if this hurts (to check the local anesthetic is working properly).
- This can sting (when you are injecting the anesthetic).
- You may feel some palpitations now. It is normal. Do not worry.
- You may feel some chest pain. It's nothing to worry about.
- You will feel a burning sensation in your head and stomach during injection of contrast material. It is also normal.
- Breathe in deeply.
- Breathe out deeply and hold your breath.

Talking to the Patient's Family

Before the Procedure

- Your father/husband/mother/wife/son/daughter is about to undergo a cardiac catheterization. Depending on findings, it will take approximately *N* minutes. The procedure does not need a general anesthetic, only local anesthesia, so your father (etc.) will remain conscious. I will let you know how the procedure went as soon as we finish.

After the Procedure

- Good news
  - Everything has gone fine from a technical point of view; we will look carefully at the images and the report will be sent to your referring physician. Your father (etc.) is doing fine. In a few minutes, you will see him. Please make sure he does not move his right leg for 8 hours.
- Bad news
  - I am afraid your father's condition is critical. He will be transferred to the ICU.
  - Unfortunately, we have not been able to cross the stenosis so the patient will be transferred to the Department of Cardiovascular Surgery where he will be operated on on an elective basis.

- There has been a serious complication. Your father is being transferred to the operating room where he will be operated on now. We
  (the surgeon and I) will inform you of the situation as soon as the
  operation is finished.

Teaching Residents

These are some of the most common commands given in interventional
cardiology suites:
- Prep the patient.
- Drape the patient.
- Make sure that the patient's groin has been shaved, scrubbed, and
  draped.
- Has the puncture site been scrubbed?
- Locate the right common femoral artery (RCFA) by palpation.
- Locate the left radial artery by palpation.
- Puncture the artery.
- Do not force the wire.
- Inject local anesthetic as deeply as possible and do not forget to aspirate
  before injecting.
- Tape the lower abdominal pannus back away from the groin.
- Nick the skin with a small blade.
- Use a hemostat to check fluoroscopically the proper position of the in-
  tended entry site.
- The skin entry must be over the lower femoral head and the puncture
  site over the medial third of the femoral head.
- Advance the needle in a single forward thrust.
- Have you flushed the cath (catheter)?
- Have you checked for free backflow?
- Do not lose the wire.
- Wipe the guidewire.
- Manipulate gently.
- Rotate in a clockwise direction.
- Counter clockwise rotation please.
- Remove the "over-the-wire."
- Inflate (deflate) the balloon at 12.
- The stent sizing is appropriate.
- The stent is patent.
- That hazy image looks like a clot.
- Let's IVUS this artery.
- Peel away the sheath.
- Introduce the catheter over the wire.
- Do not persevere with catheter manipulation.
- Try again. Do not force the wire. Rotate it gently.

- We could not cross the lesion.
- The stent has migrated into the subclavian artery. Give me a snare device.
- Dampening of blood pressure.
- Extra care must be taken with hydrophilic wires to avoid dissection.
- Retract the balloon leaving the wire across the lesion.
- Keep the balloon deflated by suctioning with a syringe.
- Let's measure the ASD diameter with the balloon. What diameter has the indentation?
- Please insert the Amplatzer within the sheath.
- Release the device.
- Look! That is an intracardiac recording from the right atrium (HRA).
- Take the ablation catheter to the site along the mitral annulus, which recorded earliest ventricular activity.
- Apply radiofrequency energy. You will see how the delta wave disappears.
- There is retrograde atrial activation.
- Please advance the mapping catheter.
- Note that the AF has a variable cycle and is self-terminating.
- Hold the ventricular lead. I will connect the pulse-generator.
- Turn on the programmer please. Let's check this pacemaker.
- Close the incision please. Continuous suture.

Talking to Nurses

- May I have my gown tied?
- Would you tie my gown?
- Tie me up, please.
- Dance with me (informal way of asking to have your gown tied).
- I'll go scrub in a minute.
- Give Dr. García a pair of shoe covers.
- Give Dr. García a thyroid shield.
- Give Dr. García a lead apron.
- Mary, I forgot my thyroid shield. Could you put one on me?
- Is the patient monitored yet?
- A phone call? Tell him I'll call back later; I can't break scrub now.
- May I have another pair of gloves, please?
- May I have a pair of lead gloves?
- We've had an iliac dissection. Page the vascular surgeon.

Talking To Technologists

- Can I have this image magnified, please?
- Could you please collimate the image? I'm burning out my body.
- An LPO 45°, please.
- Right posterior oblique. 45°.
- Film at 15 frames per second.
- Road mapping, please.
- I would like to see that lesion clearly; what projection do you suggest?

The Angiographic Equipment

- The *generator* provides the electrical energy from which X-rays are generated and contains the circuitry needed to provide a controlled and stable radiation output. The mid- to high-frequency inverter was the most popular generator design. Flat panel technology is getting widespread worldwide acceptance for its high quality and contrast saving.
- The *X-ray tube* is made of a tungsten filament cathode and a spinning anode disk with a tungsten surface. Electrons go from the cathode to the anode where they are stopped by its tungsten surface.
- The *image intensifier* converts the X-ray pattern that penetrates the patient to an intensified image. Its field of view ranges from 4 to 16 inches, depending on the magnification factor. Modern machines have a different technology with direct digital acquisition capacity.
- The *patient table* is usually made of carbon fiber to provide enough strength to support an adult patient while minimizing the attenuation of X-rays.
- The *gantry stand* contains both the X-ray tube housing with collimator and the image intensifier/imaging chain.
- The *TV or digital monitors.*
- *Contrast injectors* allow the adjustment of injection volume, peak injection rate, and acceleration to peak rate. *Contrast injector* arms can be ceiling-suspended or mounted on the table.

Some Common Standing Orders for Nursing Units

These are some of the commonest orders for nursing IC units. Non–native English-speaking interventional cardiologists must be familiar with them in order to be able to write them down on the chart.

Patient Preparation

- Premedicate with diazepam (Valium) 10 mg PO (oral intake) given on call to angiography. Reduce dose for elderly patients.
- Obtain informed consent.
- Patient must void urine before leaving the ward for the cath lab.
- Transfer the patient to the angiography suite with his/her identification plate, chart, and latest laboratory reports on chart. (New technologies allow having access to the complete history of the patient from computers everywhere at the hospital).
- Clear fluids only after midnight (for morning appointment).
- Clear fluids only after breakfast (for afternoon appointment).
- Insert Foley catheter.
- Vigorous hydration (NSS at 125 ml/h)
- Prophylactic antibiotics IV
- Establish a peripheral IV.

Postprocedure Management

- Bed rest for 8 h, with puncture site evaluation.
- Vigorous hydration until oral intake is adequate.
- Stop analgesics and remove Foley catheter 24 h after the procedure.
- Follow-up chest X-rays in 24 h.

Chart entries following interventional procedures would be a SOAP note as described elsewhere. In addition, a description of the procedure, as simple as possible, should include the doctors' name, the patient ID, the employed material, anatomic and hemodynamic findings, and the outcome of the procedure.

For contrast reactions, a form rather than chart entry is used. The information is similar and includes:

- Type and volume of contrast given
- Type and severity of reaction
- Action taken
- Future recommendation

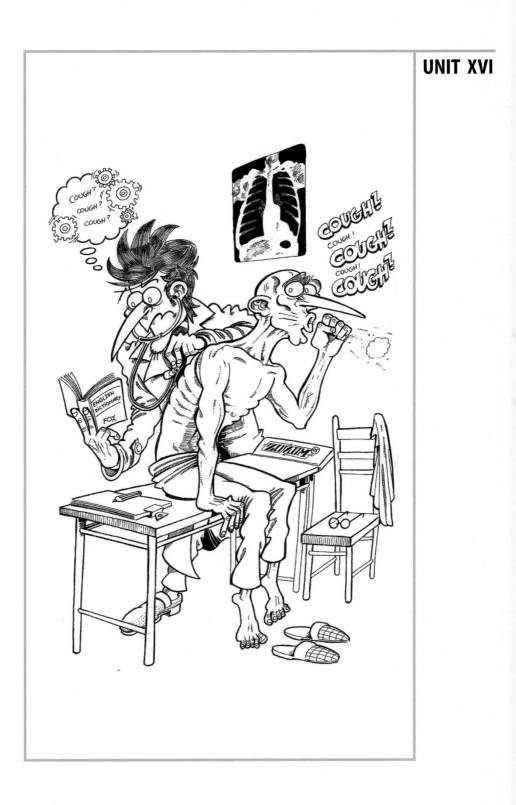

Unit XVI   Electrocardiogram Interpretation

Introduction

This chapter is not intended to be a comprehensive guide to EKG interpretation (ECG in UK English), and we are aware that the concepts we talk about are extremely basic for a cardiology resident, let alone a cardiologist. In the following lines, we want to get used with the language of this basic cardiologic tool: the electrocardiogram. Although all non–native English speaking cardiologists can perfectly understand what they read about EKGs it is quite likely that they do not feel at ease talking and writing about it.

The EKG tracing below shows the labeling of the EKG waveforms (Fig. XVI.1).

By following the Dubin textbook (*Rapid Interpretation of EKGs*. D. Dubin, 2000, Cover Publishing Company, ISBN-13: 9780912912066) stepwise mode of interpretation, every EKG tracing must be evaluated according to eight steps:

1. Rate

    The first step is to determine the Rate, which can be eyeballed by means of the following technique. Locate the QRS complex that is closest to a

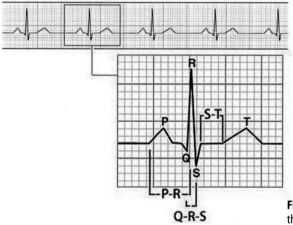

Fig. XVI.1. EKG tracing showing the waveforms and complexes

dark vertical line. Then count either forward or backwards to the next QRS complex. For each vertical line you pass, select the next number off the mnemonic "300-150-100-75-60-50" to estimate the rate in beats per minute (BPM).

In other words, if you pass two lines before the next QRS, the heart rate (HR) would be less than 150. Remember that this is merely an estimate. You should use real measurements to determine the exact HR (for precise measurement: each large box represents 200 ms and small boxes represent 40 ms).

2. Rhythm

After the determination of the rate, we determine both the regularity and the source of the rhythm. The prime concern is whether the source of the rhythm is the SA (sinoatrial) node or an ectopic pacemaker. To determine whether the source of the rhythm is the "sinus" or an ectopic rhythm, you need to look at the relationship of the P wave, if present, with the QRS complex.

We must also look at the quality and quantity of P waves before each QRS. There should only be one P wave before each QRS. The P wave should be in only one direction, and not biphasic (except for leads V_1 and V_2). It should also be closer than 200 ms to the QRS. The shape of the P wave should also be gently rounded and not peaked.

3. Axis

To do this we need to understand the basic 6 leads and their geometry. The EKG waveform comes from a measurement of surface voltages between 2 leads. A wave that is traveling towards the positive (+) lead will inscribe an upwards deflection of the EKG; conversely, a wave traveling away from the positive lead will inscribe a downward deflection. Waves that are traveling at a 90° angle to a particular lead will create no deflection and are called an isoelectric lead.

The axis is a single electrical vector, sum of the all the vectors produced by the EKG. This summed vector should in general be pointing to the same direction (down-left) for a normal heart; this makes sense if we think about the electrical conduction system of the heart which sends a signal from de SA node (top right) to the Purkinje fibers (bottom left).

There are some tricks to save you time, but first think about a normal EKG plot; in a normal EKG both leads I and AVF will be positive as the signal travels from the SA node (top right of the heart) to the tip of the ventricles (bottom left of the heart). This is a normal axis, and leads us to the rule of thumb, if I and AVF are positive, then the axis is normal. Nonetheless, the normal axis actually allows the signal to travel up to 30° above the x-axis and 30° to the left of the y-axis.

4. Precordial leads

Understanding the precordial leads and how they align with the heart is critical for the interpretation of the EKG. First of all, let us remember how the heart is located in the chest. Note that it sits flat above the diaphragm on the left side of the chest, and is pointed slightly to the left. The precordial leads correlate to the actual heart anatomy.

V_1–V_2 are over the right ventricle, while V_4–V_6 are over the left ventricle. V_3 is a transitional lead, and is approximately over the intraventricular septum, so it covers some of the electrical activity of both ventricles. Remember that the bulk of the left ventricle is posterior, so feel free to create a V_7 and V_8 to get more information of the left ventricle.

5. Hypertrophy

   Hypertrophy is the increase in size of the myocardial myocytes leading to thicker walls. It can be non-pathological, as in the case of people who frequently perform isometric exercise such as the lifting of heavy weights in which the straining and Valsalva maneuvers produce an increased afterload.

   Extending this thought, we can see how hypertrophy can occur in the pathological sense by thinking about increased afterload on the heart as in individuals with high blood pressure, which causes a left sided afterload increase.

   We need to examine both ventricles for evidence of hypertrophy there. Since increased muscle mass, logically leads to an increase in the signal, we would expect to see changes in the QRS complex morphology. For right ventricular hypertrophy, we look at V_1, and less at V_2 and V_3. For Left ventricular hypertrophy you will have a large S wave in V_1 and a large R wave in V_5.

6. Blocks

   A block is an interruption of the normal flow of an electrical impulse traveling down from the SA node to the ventricles. The block can occur in the SA and atrioventricular (AV) nodes as well as in the bundles.

   a. SN block

      It is a failure of the sinus node to transmit an impulse, and is usually seen as a complete pause of 1 beat.

   b. AV node block

      It is a block that delays the electrical impulse between the atria and the ventricles in the AV node.

      i. First-degree AV block

         The PR interval greater than 0.2 s.

      ii. Second-degree AV block

         There is more than one P wave preceding each QRS complex.

      iii. Third-degree AV block.

         It is a complete block of signals from the atria to the ventricles. The lack of synchronization is what determines whether you are in a second-degree AV block with a greater than 1:1 ratio, or a third degree.

c. Bundle branch blocks (BB)

BB are blocks within the ventricular bundles, and normally consist of a left or right bundle branch block. It can be of the entire ventricular bundle or a fascicle of a given bundle. The key to recognize a bundle block is to find an R–R wave and a QRS wider than 0.12 s.

7. Ischemia, Infarct, Injury

The ST segment is most often affected in ischemic conditions. The hallmark of acute myocardial ischemia is the elevation of ST segment. After the ischemia has progressed to an infarct the EKG will show an inverted T wave. A pronounced Q wave and loss of all or part of the R wave may also present.

Subendocardial ischemia is represented on the EKG as ST-segment depression.

8. Miscellaneous

a. Ventricular fibrillation

Often call "v-fib," it is the most life-threatening arrhythmia, and is often the end rhythm before the asystole of death. The EKG pattern of v-Fib is recognized by a total lack of organized activity, ranging from coarse (large amplitude) to fine (close to asystole) in amplitude.

b. Tachycardia

Like any other heart rhythm, the origin of the signal can be either atrial or ventricular. The most common cause of pathologic tachycardias results from re-entry.

c. Digitalis toxicity

Digitalis is a very old cardiac drug derived from the foxglove plant. Digitalis overdose can have effects ranging from mild 1° AV block to junctional rhythms through fatal arrhythmias. The most noticeable change to the EKG is the "swooping" ST-segment depression.

d. Hyperkalemia

The most prominent feature of an EKG of a hyperkalemic patient is the peaked T wave. The other feature of the hyperkalemic EKG is a stretching of entire waveform.

EKG Jargon

- Mean electrical axis
- Counterclockwise rotation
- Clockwise rotation
- Leftward or rightward axis deviation
- Septal forces
- Vectoral summation
- Limb and precordial leads
- Frontal axis

- Horizontal axis
- Biphasic P wave
- Heart rate
- P mitrale; notched P wave
- P pulmonale; P congenitale; peaked P wave
- ST–T changes
- "Current of injury"
- Reciprocal ST-segment displacement
- ST-segment elevation convex upward
- Reciprocal changes
- QS pattern; QR pattern
- R-wave voltage
- Dropped beats
- Conduction delay
- Right or left bundle branch block
- Atrial premature beats
- LASFB: Left anterior-superior fascicular block
- LPFB: Left posterior fascicular block
- Left septal fascicle
- Bifascicular block
- Trifascicular block (bilateral bundle-branch block)
- Preexcitation
- Accessory pathway (James, Brechenmacher, Mahaim, Kent bundles)
- Wolff-Parkinson-White syndrome
- Lown-Ganong-Levine syndrome
- Delta wave (initial slurring of the QRS complex)
- LV strain (ST-segment depression with T-wave inversion in leads over the left ventricle)
- Intrinsicoid deflection
- Long Q–T interval
- R-on-T phenomenon
- Early repolarization pattern
- U wave

Talking to Other Cardiologists about EKGs

Case 1
- Good morning Dr. Johnson. Would you please help me with this EKG?
- *Of course Dr. Lewis. Let's see. ... It is a sinus rhythm tracing with a normal axis; I don't see any conduction abnormalities, but it seems to me that the ST-segment is a little bit elevated. What are the patient's symptoms?*
- He complains of typical chest pain.
- *When did the pain start?*
- A few days ago. He has a fever and cough.

- *Well, Dr. Lewis. I think we have a diagnosis made. It is not an acute coronary syndrome because the ST-changes are widespread through all precordial and limb leads. Otherwise, according to patient symptoms it seems to me that your patient could have a pericarditis. Let's perform an ultrasound scan.*

Case 2
- Dr. Di Mario, what do you think about this rhythm?
- *Well my dear colleague; you always challenge us with interesting cases. As you can see, there is no P wave before this QRS complex, but it is present in the rest of the tracing.*
- Yes you're right. My first thought was an SN block. But don't you think it is just an artifact? Take a careful look and you will see the P wave in V$_2$.
- *Nope! Dr. Lakeside, I'm afraid that the artifact is that "P wave" you see in V$_2$.*
- OK. Let's look for the chairman. He will surely help us.

Case 3
- Dr. Leon, I have a shocked patient in bay 4. Could you look at the monitor with me please?
- *It's always a pleasure to help you, Dr. Wellington.*
- Thanks. Look: this is a 75-year-old man who was found unconscious on the floor. The ambulance has transferred him to our facility in just 5 minutes. Do you think it is a VT?
- *Taking into account the wideness of the QRS as the only parameter, it could be a VT. However, it has an irregular pattern, it has a right bundle branch block, and there isn't retrograde conduction. Did you have a 12-lead EKG done?*
- Not yet, I have only some EKG strips available. But I think you are right. It seems more an AF with abnormal conduction instead of a VT. Thank you very much Dr. Leon.

Case 4
- Hey! Hello, I'm Jessie Smith. I'm the first-year resident of Intensive Care. You are a cardiology resident, aren't you?
- *Yes, I am. Pleased to meet you. Why are you so disturbed?*
- My boss is gone to the cafeteria for a while and I've got a problem with this patient. Do you see what I mean?
- *Asystole!!! Flat line on the monitor. START CPR!!!!! (laughing out loud)*
- What is that so funny, Doctor?
- *The patient is completely awake and the same monitor shows a normal BP. Don't worry Dr. Smith. It is just that someone has disconnected the EKG electrodes.*

Describing EKG Findings

At some institutions, there is one cardiologist that reads the EKGs that are done in other services (external consultation, pre-anesthesia, etc.). There are some word order and description rules that must be used to send a clear message to the physician that will evaluate the patient.

How to Report an EKG

Description is followed by interpretation. The description typically is:

1. Rhythm
2. Conduction intervals
3. Cardiac axis
4. Description of the QRS complexes
5. Description of the ST segments and T waves
6. Description of abnormalities as described above

A report of a normal EKG would be as follows:

- Sinus rhythm, (rate/per minute according to age and other things)
- PR interval normal (around 0.08 s)
- QRS duration normal, according to rate/per minute. It may be normal around 0.06 (more or less), but 0.06 s will be always abnormal.
- Normal cardiac axis (around 50–70°)
- Normal QRS complexes
- Normal T waves

Case 1
Normal sinus rhythm. Frequency 75 bpm. Electrical axis at 75°. Normal PR interval (0.14 s). Abnormal QRS duration (0.18 s) with morphology of right bundle branch block and T-wave inversion in right precordial leads. Premature ventricular ectopic beat.

Describing Holter Monitoring (24-h EKG Recording)

Holter (24-h EKG) monitoring is a procedure to record for 24 continuous hours of several leads of the EKG on an individual patient. This is accomplished by attaching a miniature electronic tape recording device with several lead wires attached to the patient's chest over the heart. The complete report includes some pages that describe the information, as suggested:

First page:

- Patient's data
- Minimal, average, and maximal heart rates

- Number of pauses between heart beats
- Number of abnormal ventricular and supraventricular (atrial or nodal) events (beats).
- Abnormal movements of the baseline of the EKG (ST segment) are reported.

Page 2 of the report indicates the following:

1. The time of the events.
2. The total beats with the minimal, maximal and average.
3. The total ventricular events with the number of couplets (two successive such beats in a row).
4. The number of triplets (three successive beats in a row) with the time of each. The number of runs of these ventricular, abnormal beats of three or more (defined as ventricular tachycardia) are also given.
5. The number of beats in these runs per hour.

In addition, the abnormal atrial and/or nodal (supraventricular) beats are analyzed as to total per hour, number of couplets, number of runs of supraventricular tachycardia (at rates of a 100 or more per minute) are reported.

Similarly, runs of bradycardia (with heart rates of 60/min or below are totaled, and timed abnormal pauses between heart beats are recorded as to number time and duration in seconds. The atrial to ventricular rate ratio is presented as well (normally 1:1).

The third page presents graphics of above events as to the number and time of occurrence.

The fourth page represents a graph of the heart rate versus time, as well as the status of the baseline in relationship to the ST segment.

Pages 5 and 6 delineate the hourly activities and complaints of the patient.

Pages 6, 7, and 8 give samples of the recorded EKG strips from various positions (V_5, V_2, V_3) on the patient's chest. You can add footnotes to describe important findings (i.e., Note the premature supraventricular (atrial) beats (S) at 14:01 and 15:58 hours.)

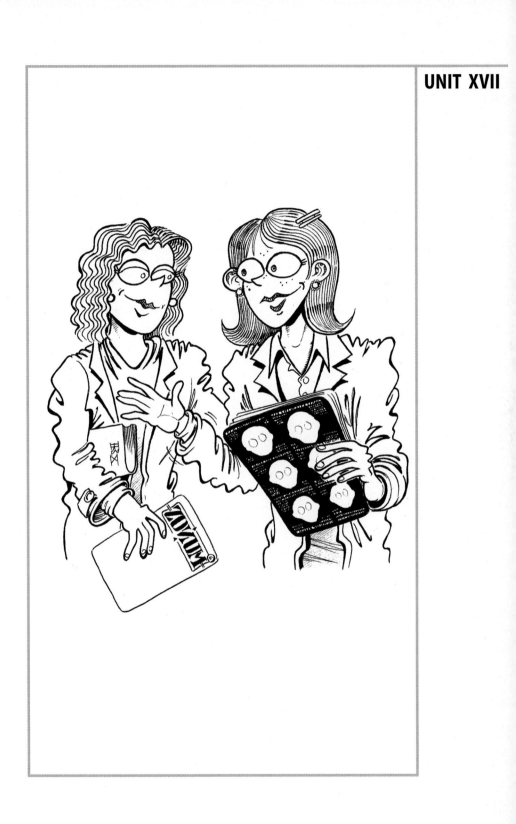

Unit XVII   Heart Transplantation

Introduction

One of the most exciting situations that a cardiologist can face-up is heart transplantation. On the one hand, the patient with heart failure and his/her family that are desperately waiting for a new heart coming from a human donor need a precise and accurate information on the entire procedure, and it is precisely the cardiologist the one who is supposed to provide it. On the other hand, the family of the donor and many health care professionals involved in the transplant protocol must be informed thoroughly.

This unit aims to help non–native English speaking cardiologists who have to talk to colleagues, patients, and patients' families in an extremely difficult scenario. It is not easy to talk about death, donors, last will, etc., and it is not easy either to give the correct information to an anxious and sometimes dyspneic patient who is about to be operated on on an emergent basis.

After the operation, the follow-up of a heart transplant recipient is plenty of tests, medication, immunosupression secondary effects, biopsies, coronary graft vasculopathy, etc. It is an extensive language field in which non–native English speakers must be as fluent as possible in order to be able to convey accurate information.

Current Transplant Jargon

- Autologous: From the same person
- Grafting: synonymous of transplantation; replacement of a failing organ or tissue by a functioning one
- Allograft: graft from the same species
- Xenotransplant: from a different species
- Antigens: substances that cause the immune system to react to foreign materials
- Donor and recipient
- HLA types (human leukocyte antigen)
- Heart transplantation
- Graft rejection

- Donated organs
- Donor card
- Postmortem organ procurement
- Cross-match
- Cyclosporine-A
- Tacrolimus
- Prednisone
- Brain-dead donor
- Allocation system
- Organ transplant laws
- Ethical concerns
- Graft-versus-host disease
- Immunosuppressant drugs
- Allocation score
- Post-transplant lymphoproliferative disorder
- Endomyocardial biopsy
- Acute rejection protocol
- Chronic rejection
- Coronary vasculopathy
- Myocardial performance
- Ejection fraction
- Diastolic function
- Ventricular assist device
- Graft failure
- Re-transplantation
- Immune response
- Xenograft
- Organ donation
- Donor consent
- Presumed consent
- Brain-dead statutes
- Non-invasive graft-rejection diagnosis
- Organ waiting list
- Panel reactive antibodies (PRA)
- Mechanical pump assist
- Coronary allograft vascular disease
- End-stage heart disease
- Compatible donor
- Universal donor
- Hyperacute reaction
- Cardiac output
- Antiviral drugs

Talking about Brain Death (to the Donor's Family)

Hacker slang terminology uses the "brain-death" expression to design failure rather than malfunctioning, or simple stupidity. However, in our working scenario, brain death normally refers to a state of irreversible destruction of the brain.

The doctor, who must explain this condition to the donor's family, should be fluent, sensible, and confident enough to reassure them and, at the same time, help them to solve this challenging situation.

- Mr. and Mrs. Smith, I am so sorry for this. We have made every possible effort to save John's life, but the accident was terrible and his head was almost crushed, as you saw. He's been declared brain dead according to our hospital's ethical committee and national laws regarding transplantation fields.
- Brain death applies to the situation when the heart continues to beat, with the breathing maintained mechanically after the brain has permanently ceased to function.
- Under natural conditions when the brain ceases to function, breathing immediately stops, and soon after this, the heart stops beating due to lack of oxygen. If breathing is taken over by a mechanical ventilator, oxygenation is maintained and the heart can continue to beat, for days at least, because the heart muscle acts on its own independently of the brain.
- We found a "donor card" within John's clothes, and we would like to inform you of this important wish. We have a very young patient with an end-stage heart disease, included in the organ-awaiting list a few months ago, that is compatible with John's HLA system.
- Mrs. Marshall, I'd like to introduce you to Mrs. Jones. She is one of the social workers at our hospital and will be in charge of everything regarding John's burial and anything else you may need. We are truly grateful for your cooperation. For ethical reasons we cannot give you data from the recipient, but you can be sure that he and his family will be forever grateful.

Talking to the Recipient before the Operation

- Jane, we have a heart that is compatible with your immune system. Finally, you will be operated on. Now we are preparing the OR. The nurse will come to give you some instructions and prepare you for the operation. Do not worry. Everything will be OK.
- Your family is coming. Your relatives are on their way to the hospital now.
- Let me briefly explain the procedure:

- A specialist in cardiovascular anesthesia will give you general anesthesia. So you will not be aware of anything and will not suffer any pain at all.
- Intravenous antibiotics are given to prevent bacterial wound infections. We have already started the infusion.
- After the cardiopulmonary bypass is started and adequate blood circulation is established, your diseased heart is removed.
- The donor heart is attached to your blood vessels.
- After the blood vessels are connected, your new heart is warmed up and will begin beating.
- Then, you are taken off from the heart/lung machine.
- Your new heart is stimulated to maintain a regular beat with medications for two to five days after surgery, until the new heart functions normally on its own.
- Once stabilized, you will be transferred from the ICU to the Cardiology ward.

Talking to the Patient's Family

Before the procedure, you must explain the same issues described above to the patient's family: "Your father/husband/mother/wife/son/daughter is about to undergo the operation we all have been waiting for …"
After the procedure, there are two possibilities:

- Good news:
  - Everything has gone well from a technical point of view; we will be around and take care of him carefully. In a few minutes you will see your father (etc.) He is doing fine. Please follow the visit schedule shown in the ICU door.
- Bad news:
  - I am afraid your father's condition is critical. Unfortunately, we had some serious complications with the coagulation system and he needs to be re-operated on now. We will inform you of the situation as soon as the operation is finished.

Leaving the Hospital

- Well, Mrs. Townsend, your heart has regained its normal function, meaning the heart pumps a normal amount of blood to the rest of your body.
- You will notice that your heart beats slightly faster than normal because its nerves have been cut during surgery.

- You will notice as well that your new heart also does not increase its rate as quickly during exercise. Don't worry about that. You will feel much better, and your capacity for exercise will be dramatically improved.
- You can return to work in less than 3 months from now, and you will be progressively able to do other daily activities.
- We have already talked about medication. Should you have any problem or concern, do not hesitate to contact us.

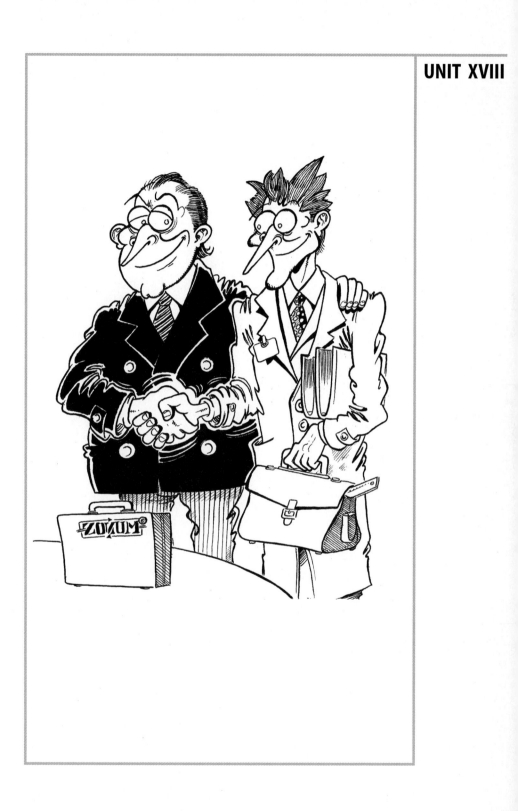

Unit XVIII   Clinical Session

Introduction

Residents and fellows during their initial training years learn how to present patients to a mixed audience of clinicians and surgeons, who will decide the best treatment approach. In cardiovascular medicine, it is routine to discuss the best course of treatment for a patient with coronary disease, valve abnormality, vascular disease, or congenital defect. In a non-emergent situation, because the session can be prepared for, non–native English speaking doctors can make very good clinical presentations if they learn some communication skills mentioned elsewhere in this book.

Presenting a Case

Every hospital, and each department director, has its/his/her own preferences regarding the way a clinical case must be presented. We present three vascular cases. In these sessions, controversial approaches to patient treatment are typical; the way the fellow presents the case will influence final the decision(s).

Case presentation 1

Dr. Ponce (fellow): Good morning every one. This is the first case of today's session.

Dr. Wellens (clinical consultant): Just a sec, Dr. Ponce. Any emergencies last night?

Dr. Ponce: Yes, boss. One 87-year-old female admitted for cardiogenic shock, and she didn't make it. Nothing else worth mentioning.

Dr. Wellens: Thank you, Doctor. Please go ahead with the first case.

Dr. Ponce: Well, this is a 57-year-old man, a postal carrier, who came to consultation complaining of calf pain induced by walking more than 100 m. He is a heavy smoker, and his blood cholesterol has been high for

2 years. He does not want to take any medication and is trying to control it with low-fat diet. No known allergies, and there aren't previous medical or surgical disorders. Since 2 months ago, he notices severe right calf pain when walking more than 300 m (2 blocks). Pain is relieved by rest. As a postal carrier, this affects his livelihood, and he is concerned about the symptom.

Dr. Wellens: Well, OK. What about physical findings?

Dr. Ponce: Normal BP. Normal heart sounds without murmurs. Right limb: bruit over right femoral artery. Artery pulsations present, including the foot arteries. Left limb: bruit over left femoral artery. Femoral artery pulses present. No popliteal or distal pulses.

Dr. Nabel (surgical consultant): Have you got an EKG for this patient?

Dr. Ponce: Sure. The electrocardiogram shows regular sinus rhythm. When evaluating the QRS complex, one can see clear Q waves in derivation II, III, and AVF. These Q waves are showing an old inferior infarction. The repolarization is atypical. One can see, in different derivations, flat T waves with the ST segment just less than 1 mm under the zero line. I think they are non-specific, but the Q waves in the derivation II, III, and AVF are typical of an old inferior infarction.

Dr. Wellens: What is your next step in light of this patient condition?

Dr. Ponce: There clearly is a problem with this man. The EKG is abnormal, and the vascular findings are clearly clinically abnormal. So just reassuring him would not be the right thing to do. He needs to be examined to determine the magnitude of the problem. Thus, the examination should be non-invasive, and the best way to approach this is to measure ankle pressure. There is at this time no need for duplex scanning, as it describes the anatomy present. It is much too early to perform contrast angiogram. This should only be carried out when an invasive treatment is one of the possibilities (and this is not yet the case).

Dr. Wellens: Which data do we have? What treatment does he now need?

Dr. Ponce: The ankle pressures and the gradients measured are clearly abnormal, so something should be done for him. Normally the pressure gradient, which is ankle/arm, is 1 or more, with the lowest value at 0.9. Here it is down to 0.58; thus, it is clearly abnormal. Treatment is necessary in such a patient. Drugs and Exercise! Exercise to improve the claudication. Drugs can eventually help with the claudication too, but primarily they are used to reduce atherothrombotic ischemic events such as myocardial infarction and stroke. Note, interventional treatment, such as percutaneous transluminal angioplasty (PTA) or vascular surgery, is not yet necessary.

Dr. Wellens: Any comments Dr. Nabel? Doctors?

Dr. Nabel and colleagues: Nope! I do agree with the proposed treatment approach.

Case presentation 2

Dr. Ponce: Male, 58 years old, whose presenting complaint is, "My right calf cramps whenever I walk a quarter of a mile uphill." The symptom's been present for 2 months. Mr. Smith's medical history includes a myocardial infarction at age 53; hypertension, 8 years; type II diabetes mellitus, 4 years. He smoked 2 packs a day for 35 years. Medications include captopril and glyburide (glibenclamide).

Dr. Nabel: Physical findings?

Dr. Ponce: Lungs: clear to palpation and auscultation. Heart: S4, no murmurs. Abdomen: right lower quadrant bruit, no masses. Extremities: diminished right femoral pulse, absent right popliteal and pedal pulses; normal left femoral, popliteal, and pedal pulses.

Dr. Nabel: What are the relevant diagnoses?

Dr. Ponce: Mr. Smith is a typical patient with systemic atherothrombosis. There are multiple clinical manifestations of this problem. Foremost, he has peripheral arterial disease (PAD). This is manifested in his history by symptoms of classic intermittent claudication – his calf cramps when he walks a hill – and the physical examination reveals abnormal pulses. In addition, the patient had a prior MI, indicative of coronary artery disease. He also has extracranial cerebrovascular disease – a carotid bruit was heard on physical examination. This patient has high BP, type II diabetes mellitus, and hypercholesterolemia. As is often the case in patients with atherothrombosis, there is more than one risk factor. In summary, he has systemic atherothrombosis. He has multiple clinical manifestations of this problem and multiple risk factors, including PAD, coronary artery disease (prior MI), carotid bruit (asymptomatic), hypertension, type II diabetes mellitus, and hypercholesterolemia.

Dr. Allegra (non-presenting fellow): So, what the next step should be?

Dr. Ponce: Segmental pressure measurements. This non-invasive test enables us to determine the presence of peripheral arterial stenosis, assess their severity, and gain insight into their location. Pulse-volume recordings are often used as an adjunctive test with segmental pressure measurements. An abnormal pulse-volume recording distal to the stenosis provides further evidence of PAD. Many laboratories use duplex ultrasonography of the leg to assess PAD. However, it requires considerable time to perform this procedure and the information gained does not necessarily increase the knowledge of the presence or severity of PAD. Magnetic resonance angiogram is a test that can be used to demonstrate the anatomy of the peripheral vasculature. The technology is improving, as is its resolution. However, at this time MRA is not indicated for the routine evaluation of PAD, but may be employed in patients who will ultimately be considered for revascularization procedures. Contrast arteriography is rarely if ever necessary for diagnostic purposes. It is performed, however, when interventions such as PTA or reconstructive surgery are being considered. Am I right Dr. Wellens?

Dr. Wellens: Yes doctor. What you say is in accordance with the guidelines recently published in the *Journal of Vascular Surgery*.

Case presentation 3

Dr. Holmes (Presenting fellow): The patient is Mr. Björk, a 62 year-old gentleman with diabetes and hypertension. He has never smoked. The patient has a previous history of CABG in 1985. Over the past few months, he has had several episodes of hospitalization for congestive heart failure. The patient did not have chest pain or dyspnea with exertion. However, he stated that his left knee would hurt with walking more than one to two city blocks, but would be relieved with stopping for a couple of minutes. He also reported an episode of right facial numbness 2 weeks ago that lasted less than 5 minutes.

Dr. García (cardiologist): Any other test to assess his actual heart condition?

Dr. Holmes: A stress thallium test demonstrated lateral ischemia with nonsustained ventricular tachycardia at a low workload. Cardiac catheterization revealed 100% proximal occlusion of the LAD, left circumflex artery, and RCA. LIMA-LAD, SVG–RCA, and SVG–lateral branch of the Lat Cx were all patent (though the vein grafts had moderate atheroma throughout); however, there was severe, diffuse distal disease beyond the touchdown of all three grafts. Additionally, there was a discrete 75% stenosis immediately beyond the anastomosis of the SVG to Lat Cx. The patient was referred to our center as an outpatient for further management.

Dr. Wellens (vascular consultant): And what about that knee pain?

Dr. Holmes: Lower extremity pain in an older patient could be due to multiple causes. The history and physical examination are helpful, though often over time there is a need for non-invasive testing to differentiate among musculoskeletal, neurological, and vascular causes. While arthritis is a possibility, in this case of a man with diabetes, hypertension, and extensive coronary artery disease, claudication should be considered in the differential diagnosis.

Dr. Wellens: What is the most likely cause of the right facial numbness?

Dr. Holmes: Transient ischemic attack is the most likely explanation. The episode did not last long enough to be considered a stroke. Seizure is a possibility worth considering, but is not high on the differential. While people with diabetes are at increased risk of neuropathy, this transient episode of facial numbness is an unlikely manifestation of neuropathy.

Dr. Wellens: What are the appropriate studies to order?

Dr. Holmes: Carotid ultrasound would be important to look for carotid artery stenosis. Echocardiography would be necessary to assess left ventricular function, perhaps also to screen for embolic sources. PVRs would also be important to assess for peripheral vascular disease; importantly, the presence of palpable distal pulses does not exclude the diagnosis of peripheral arterial disease.

Dr. Wellens: Well done Dr. Holmes. Please ask for those tests and we'll see the results in tomorrow's session. Thanks a lot.

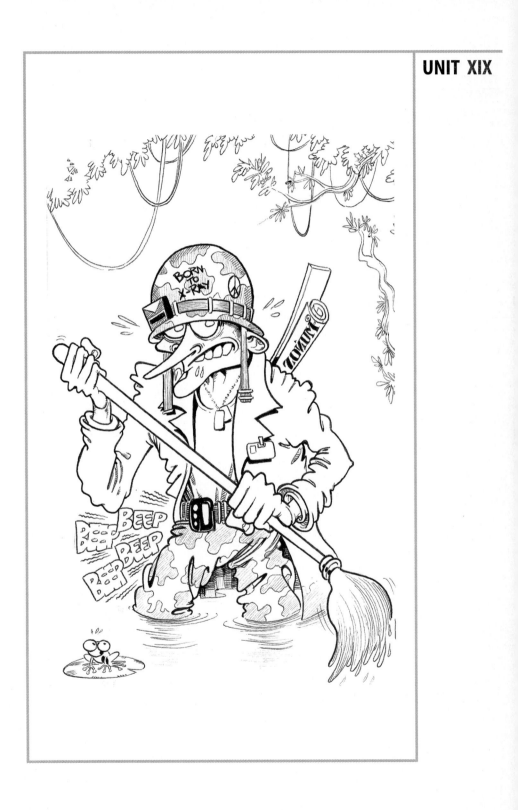

Unit XIX   On Call

Introduction

"Bob walked into the living room with his hand over his heart, as if he was planning on doing a quick pledge of allegiance. 'I have chest pains' was what he said, though 'I think it could be indigestion'."

This is Bob's wife explaining to you, the cardiologist on-call, what happened at home just a few minutes ago. She continues:

"So what exactly do you do when your husband announces, out of the blue, that he's having chest pains that might be indigestion? This is what came to mind in the space of a second: Make chamomile tea, get him some Mylanta, get a taxi to the hospital, call 911. As I headed to the kitchen to put water on for tea, he announced new developments. 'The pain is worse and I'm sweating.' I dialed 911."

We have previously developed, in units XI, XII, and XIII the way you should act to obtain a good clinical history with quick and smart questions. The emergency room scenario does not normally permit a quiet interview; patients and relatives are usually overexcited, and doctors, nurses, and paramedics are busy (or should be, at least). Let us follow Bob's-wife description:

"Within what seemed like seconds, the fire department showed up at our door. Four, perhaps five hunks in full gear tromped through our living room carrying axes, walkie-talkies, and oxygen. They surrounded Bob, taking his vitals and getting information from me. They told me they were going to give first aid until EMS (emergency medical service) showed up. EMS personnel were two men who immediately hooked Bob up to a portable EKG machine and determined that it was a heart attack. I looked at Bob and suddenly, in a kind of slow motion, his eyes rolled up and then closed and he slowly slumped sideways on the sofa. The portable ECG machine is also a portable defibrillator. Within seconds, Bob was sputtering back to life, arms flailing as if he were fighting off death itself."

Describing a real case is the best way to get involved. As a cardiologist/cardiology resident, you probably will never participate in ambulance-rescue procedures. But if so, and your language is not fluent enough, it is better to stay quiet and to obey orders that you surely will understand. American and British hospitals have much to do with those you see on TV series.

Let us keep on reading Bob's wife description of the arrival of her husband to the ER:

"EMS paramedics wheeled Bob in, calling out his status in their medical shorthand as a swarm of activity formed around him, 'Male, MI, post-arrest.' The emergency staff looked at Bob, incredulous. 'Post–cardiac arrest?' one of them asked. It was true. Bob looked remarkably healthy for someone who had just cheated death by a hairbreadth."

The rest of the story is your daily job: clinical diagnosis, treatment approach, and information to relatives.

Let us now make a special mention to someone that is like a keystone in the ER work: the ER unit clerks. A good unit clerk makes the ER run like a well-oiled machine. They have to be like an octopus, juggling several tasks at the same time all the while answering the constantly ringing phones. When you fill in their job for short periods here and there, you have to say if "I was forced to do it for more than an hour or two, someone would die." They are the usually under-paid and many times underappreciated unsung heroes of the ER.

Common On-Call Sentences

We have tried to compile as many "call terms, sentences, and collocations" as possible in just a few conversations. These sentences do not needs translation or any further comments and any intermediate-level English-speaking cardiologist can understand them easily provided they are within the appropriate context. Read the sentences aloud and do not let them catch you off guard.

- A pager goes off.
- The interventionalist is Q4 or Q5.
- In your next golden weekend...
- Post-call days.
- I've just reviewed your patient's EKG, and wanted to discuss the findings with you.
- I would like to obtain more information on her presentation and past surgical history.
- Thank you for contacting me regarding Mrs. Doubtfire's CT.
- I concur with the previous report.
- The next study of choice would be ...
- ER physician
- To order a coronary CT,...
- Diagnosed with ...
- Admitted for chest pain
- Admitted for oncologic work up
- Is Mr. Smith having neurological symptoms?
- To obtain it as a "next available" study, ...

- It is not emergent.
- I'll contact the technologist.
- Resident finishing call.
- Resident coming on call.
- There are two studies pending.
- POD #10 (postoperative day).
- Patient's medical record number #####.
- In the ICU on D10.
- The contact person for the patient is Dr. Ruiz.
- Her pager number is #####.
- The nurse has called for the patient.
- Transport is on the way.
- I'll follow up on these studies.
- To page the referring physician,…
- I'm the cardiologist on call.
- I want to inform you about the findings.
- I am returning a page. How can I help you?
- My pager is not working properly. May I have some fresh batteries?
- Is the patient under contact precautions?
- Is the patient intubated?
- Can the patient be repositioned in the left lateral decubitus position?
- I will get some extra help to move the patient.
- I will set up the ultrasound machine.
- Fiona was signing out to Amy.
- DNR patient
- I'm on again tonight.
- I get the weekend off.
- I'll be post-call on Tuesday and Friday.
- From then on, it's "only" every third night for the rest of the month.
- I got only one hit.
- I am scheduled to be on with …
- I've woken up from my pre-call sleep.
- "Call a code!"
- CAC in the emergency room (clear all corridors).
- It seems like every walk-in needs a brain CT.
- That make me suspicious of …
- The IV (line) has fallen out.
- We must replace the IV line.
- Everybody was either pre-call or post-call.

Additional Call Terms

- Pre-call/post-call: day preceding or following call.
- Q: Denotes frequency of call. For example, "I am Q4" means that call is taken every 4 days.
- Golden weekend: weekend uninterrupted by call. For example, on a Q4 call schedule, a golden weekend is flanked by a Thursday and Monday call.
- Home call: call taken from home where issues resolvable by phone are done so may require returning to the hospital for issues that require personal presence.
- In-house call: person on call stays in the hospital for the duration of call.
- Night float: system of call where night coverage is assigned for several days in a row (usually on a weekly basis). The person on call works at night and is free of daytime responsibilities.

On-Call Conversations

A pager goes off. A cardiologist, a cardiac surgeon, and a radiologist are having dinner at the hospital cafeteria:

- "Whose beeper (pager) is *going off*?"
- It has to be mine; the CT technologist must have finished the brain CT I was expecting," says the radiologist, producing his pager from his lab coat right pocket.
- "Are you Q4 or Q5?"
- "I am Q4."
- "Where are you going on your next *golden weekend*, Peter?
- "I am going to Spain."
- "What are the toughest days for a cardiology resident, Sam?"
- "*Post-call* days are probably the toughest for a resident."

Cardiology resident on call, *paged by internal medicine service*:

- Cardiologist: "This is Dr. Nieminen. I am the cardiologist on call. *I am returning a page. How can I help you?*"
- Nurse: "Dr. Marco, you didn't return a page from the vascular surgeon?"
- Cardiologist: "I haven't been paged in the last couple of hours."
- Nurse: "Is your pager working properly?"
- Cardiologist: I'm afraid it's *not working properly. Do you have some fresh batteries?*"

Doing an ultrasound examination at the ICU:

- Cardiologist (speaking to the ICU nurse): "Good afternoon, I am Dr. Miller. I am here to do Mr. Smith's (patient) cardiac ultrasound. *Is the patient under contact precautions?*"
- Nurse: "Yes, patient is under contact precautions for MRSA. The yellow contact gowns and gloves are in the drawer by the entrance."
- Cardiologist: "*Is the patient intubated? Can the patient be repositioned in the left lateral decubitus position?*"
- Nurse: "Yes, patient is intubated but can be turned about 30 degrees. *I will get some extra help to move the patient.*"
- Cardiologist: "Thank you. *I will set up the ultrasound machine* in the meantime."

Cardiology resident *finishing call*, speaking to resident *coming on call*:

- Cardiologist 1: "There are two *tasks pending*. The first is an ultrasound on a *postop patient*, Mr. Davis, who is *POD #5 from a CABG*, with persistent fevers and elevated white count. The patient's *medical record number is #####*. He is located *in the ICU on 8D*. The *contact person for the patient is Dr. Concha* (the cardiac surgeon). *His pager number is ####*. The second patient is Mr. Simpson. *The cath lab nurse has already been contacted and has called for the patient. Transport is on the way.*"
- Cardiologist 2: "Thanks. *I'll follow up on these studies* and contact Dr. Concha with the results."
- Cardiologist 2 (upon performance of cardiac ultrasound): "Dr. Concha, this is Dr. Miller; *I am the cardiologist on call.* Thank you for calling back. I have done Mr. Davis' ultrasound and *wanted to inform you of the findings. There is a mild pericardial effusion ...*"

Cardiology resident on call. Cardiologist's *pager goes off*. Conversation with *ER physician* in the emergency room at 3 a.m.:

- *ER physician*: "Hello, I would like to ask for a patient evaluation. Mr. Smith, 56 year-old male, recently diagnosed of aortic stenosis and is been admitted for dizziness and stubbing chest pain."
- Cardiologist: "Have you seen any conduction abnormality on the EKG?"
- ER physician:" Not at all. He is in sinus rhythm without any disturbances."
- Cardiologist: Well, since it is not an emergency, please transfer the patient to the Cardiac Care Unit. I'll see him there as soon as possible.

Pain Scale

Here we present a pain scale. In the emergency room and when being on call, doctors frequently see patients with pain. Cardiovascular doctors too. This is a useful guide to grade the pain, an always-subjective symptom.

 0 = no pain. This is as good as it gets. Enjoy yourself!
 1 = the least perceptible pain. You can only feel it if there is nothing else going on. A bruise or contusion.
 2 = pain that you can feel if you focus on it. An abrasion, a paper cut, or a blister.
 3 = pain that you notice except when you are really busy or mentally focused on something else. A laceration, a minor muscle cramp, or a large bruise.
 4 = pain that intrudes, even when you are really busy, or enjoying something. This level of pain occurs with a bad sunburn or mild to moderate arthritis.
 5 = pain that begins to interfere with your concentration, even when you are doing something important. Fractures, during the first week or two, muscle spasms, moderate to moderately severe arthritis reach this level.
 6 = pain that begins to interfere with your enjoyment of life, and with sleep. This pain will awaken you from light sleep. Spinal stenosis, mild disk herniations, and soft tissue infections reach this level of pain.
 7 = pain that causes you to stop what you are doing, gives rise to an exclamation. Smashing your thumb with a hammer will do this. Acute, severe disk herniations, joint dislocations, and acute fractures are in this category.
 8 = pain that produces an autonomic response. This level breaks you out in a sweat, and causes an increase in blood pressure and pulse. Passing a kidney stone gets you here, about once in three stones, in my experience. Acute gout attacks, open fractures, and severe arthritis can reach this level.
 9 = pain that produces a full autonomic response plus loss of dignity. Hypertension, tachycardia, diaphoresis, crying and screaming, demands for relief. Trigeminal neuralgia, some dental abscesses, deep second-degree burns, and multiple severe open fractures are at this level.
10 = suicidal pain. This is a pain, which if you knew it would only last an hour, then go away, you would try to kill yourself because you couldn't stand it for an hour. Bowel and bladder control are lost, or forgotten. Spinal epidural hematoma or abscess reaches this level for a few hours, before the nerves lose the ability to conduct. Severe multiple trauma and total body or large area burns can reach this level.

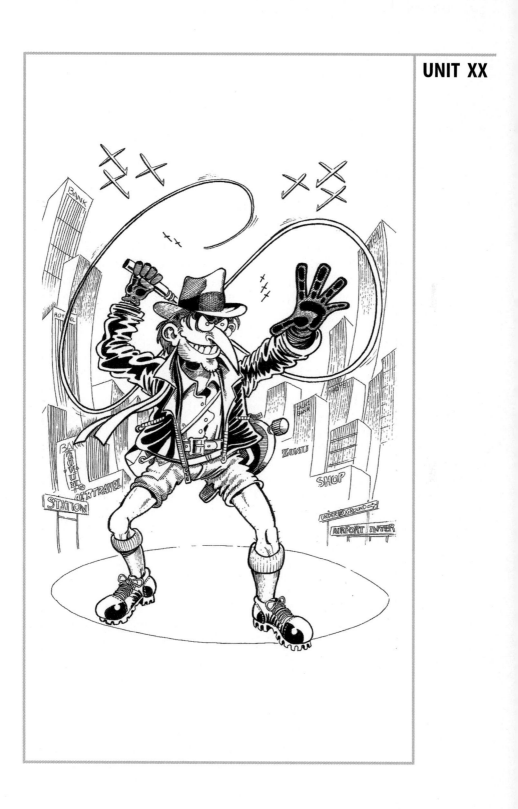

Unit XX   Conversation Survival Guide

Introduction

Fluency gives self-confidence and its lack undermines you.

The intention of this unit is not to replace conversation guides; on the contrary, we encourage you, according to your level, to use them.

Without including translations, it would have been foolish to write a conversation guide. Why, then, have we written this unit? The aim of the unit is to provide a "survival guide," a basic tool, to be reviewed by upper-intermediate speakers who are actually perfectly able to understand all the usual exchanges, but can have some difficulty in finding natural ways to express themselves in certain unusual scenarios. For instance, we are strolling with a colleague who wants us to accompany him to a jeweler's to buy a bracelet for his wife. Bear in mind that, even in your own language, fluency is virtually impossible in all situations. I have only been upset and disappointed (in English) three times. At a laundry, at an airport, and, on a third occasion, at a restaurant. I considered myself relatively fluent in English by that time but, under pressure, thoughts come to mind much faster than words and your level of fluency can be overwhelmed because of the adrenaline levels in your blood. Accept this piece of advice: Unless you are bilingual, you cannot afford to get into arguments in a language other than your own.

Many upper-intermediate speakers do not take a conversation guide when traveling abroad. They think their level is well above those who need a guide to construct basic sentences and are ashamed of being seen reading one (I myself went through this stage). I was (and they are) utterly wrong in not taking a guide because, for upper-intermediate speakers, a conversation guide has different and very important uses (as my level increased, I realized that my use of these guides changed; I did not need to read the translations, except for a few words, and I just looked for natural ways of saying things).

In my opinion, even for those who are bilingual, conversation guides are extremely helpful whenever you are in an unfamiliar environment such as, for example, a florist. How many names of flowers do you know in your own language? Probably fewer than a dozen. Think that every conversation scenario has its own jargon and a conversation guide can give you the hints that an upper-intermediate speaker may need to be actually fluent in many situations. So, do not be ashamed of carrying and reading a guide, even in public; they are the shortest way to fluency in those unfamiliar scenarios that sporadically test our English level and, what is more important, our self-confidence in English.

Whenever you have to go out to dinner, for example, review the key words and usual sentences of your conversation guide. It will not take more than 10 minutes, and your dinner will taste even better since you have ordered it with unbelievable fluency and precision. What is just a recommendable task for upper-intermediate speakers is absolutely mandatory for lower-intermediate speakers who, before leaving the hotel, should review, and rehearse the sentences they will need to ask for whatever they want to eat or, at least, to avoid ordering what they never would eat in their own country. Looking at the faces of your colleagues once the first course is served you will realize who is eating what he wanted and who, on the contrary, does not know what he ordered and, what is worse, what he is actually eating.

Let us think for a moment about this incident that happened to me when I was at the University of California, San Francisco (UCSF) Medical Center. I was invited to have lunch at a diner near the hospital, and when I asked for still mineral water, the somewhat surprised waiter answered that they did not have still mineral water but sparkling because no customer had ever asked for such a "delicacy" and offered me plain water instead. (If you do not understand this story, the important words to look up in the dictionary are diner, with one "n," still, sparkling, and plain.)

Would you be fluent without the help of a guide in a car breakdown? I did have a leak in the gas tank on a trip with my wife and mother-in-law from Boston to Niagara Falls and Toronto. I still remember the face of the mechanic in Toronto when asking me if we were staying in downtown Toronto. I answered that we were on our way back to ... Boston. I can tell you that my worn guide was vital, without it, I would not have been able to explain what the problem was. This was the last time I had to take the guide from a hidden pocket in my suitcase. Since then I have kept my guide with me, even at ... the beach, because unexpected situations may arise at any time by definition. Think of possibly embarrassing, although not infrequent, situations and ... do not forget your guide on your next trip abroad (the inside pocket of your jacket is a suitable place for those who still have not overcome the stage of "guide-ashamedness").

Those who have reached a certain level are aware of the many embarrassing situations they have had to overcome in the past to become fluent in a majority of circumstances.

Greetings

- Hi.
- Hello.
- Good morning.
- Good afternoon.
- Good evening.
- Good night.
- How are you? (Very) Well, thank you.
- How are you getting on? All right, thank you.
- I am glad to see you.
- Nice to see you (again).
- How do you feel today?
- How is your family?
- Good bye.
- Bye bye.
- See you later.
- See you soon.
- See you tomorrow.
- Give my regards to everybody.
- Give my love to your children.

Presentations

- This is Mr./Mrs. ...
- These are Mister and Misses ...
- My name is ...
- What is your name? My name is ...
- Pleased/Nice to meet you.
- Let me introduce you to ...
- I'd like to introduce you to ...
- Have you already met Mr. ...? Yes, I have.

Personal Data

- What is your name? My name is ...
- What is your surname/family name? My surname/family name is ...
- Where are you from? I am from ...
- Where do you live? I live in ...
- What is your address? My address is ...
- What is your email address? My email address is ...

- What is your phone number? My phone number is …
- What is your mobile phone/cellular number? My mobile phone/cellular number is …
- How old are you? I am …
- Where were you born? I was born in …
- What do you do? I am a radiologist.
- What do you do? I do MRI/US/CT/chest …

Courtesy Sentences

- Thank you very much. You are welcome (Don't mention it).
- Would you please …? Sure, it is a pleasure.
- Excuse me.
- Pardon.
- Sorry.
- Cheers!
- Congratulations!
- Good luck!
- It doesn't matter!
- May I help you?
- Here you are!
- You are very kind. It is very kind of you.
- Don't worry; that's not what I wanted.
- Sorry to bother/trouble you.
- Don't worry!
- What can I do for you?
- How can I help you?
- Would you like something to drink?
- Would you like a cigarette?
- I would like …
- I beg your pardon.
- Have a nice day.

Speaking in a Foreign Language

- Do you speak English/Spanish/French …? I do not speak English/Only a bit/Not a word.
- Do you understand me? Yes, I do. No, I don't.
- Sorry, I do not understand you.
- Could you speak slowly, please?
- How do you write it?
- Could you write it down?

- How do you spell it?
- How do you pronounce it?
- Sorry, what did you say?
- Sorry, my English is not very good.
- Sorry, I didn't get that.
- Could you please repeat that?
- I can't hear you.

At the Restaurant

"The same for me" is one of the most common sentences heard at tables around the world. The non-fluent English speaker links his/her gastronomic fate to a reportedly more fluent one in order to avoid uncomfortable counter-questions such as "How would you like your meat, sir?"

A simple look at a guide a few minutes before the dinner will provide you with enough vocabulary to ask for whatever you want.

Do not let your lack of fluency spoil a good opportunity to taste delicious dishes or wines.

Preliminary Exchanges

- Hello, do you have a table for three people?
- Hi, may I book a table for a party of seven for 6 o'clock?
- What time are you coming, sir?
- Where can we sit?
- Is this chair free?
- Is this table taken?
- Waiter/waitress, I would like to order.
- Could I see the menu?
- Could you bring the menu?
- Can I have the wine list?
- Could you give us a table next to the window?
- Could you give me a table on the mezzanine?
- Could you give us a table near the stage?

Ordering

- We'd like to order now.
- Could you bring us some bread, please?
- We'd like to have something to drink.
- *Here you are.*
- Could you recommend a local wine?

- Could you recommend one of your specialties?
- Could you suggest something special?
- What are the ingredients of this dish?
- I'll have a steamed lobster, please.
- *How would you like your meat, sir?*
- Rare/medium-rare/medium/well-done.
- Somewhere between rare and medium rare will be OK.
- Is the halibut fresh?
- What is there for dessert?
- *Anything else, sir?*
- No, we are fine, thank you.
- The same for me.
- *Enjoy your meal, sir.*
- *How was everything, sir?*
- The meal was excellent.
- The sirloin was delicious.
- Excuse me, I have spilled something on my tie. Could you help me?

Complaining

- The dish is cold. Would you please heat it up?
- The meat is underdone. Would you cook it a little more, please?
- Excuse me. This is not what I asked for.
- Could you change this for me?
- The fish is not fresh. I want to see the manager.
- I asked for a sirloin.
- The meal wasn't very good.
- The meat smells off.
- Could you bring the complaints book?
- This wine is off, I think. ...
- Waiter, this fork is dirty.

The Check (the Bill)

- The check, please.
- Would you bring us the check, please?
- All together, please.
- We are paying separately.
- I am afraid there is a mistake; we didn't have this.
- This is for you.
- Keep the change.

City Transportation

- I want to go to the Metropolitan Museum.
- Which bus/tram/underground line must I take for the Metropolitan?
- Which bus/tram/underground line can I take to get to the Metropolitan?
- Where does the number [...] bus stop?
- Does this bus go to ...?
- How much is a single ticket?
- Three tickets, please.
- Where must I get off for ...?
- Is this seat occupied/vacant?
- Where can I get a taxi?
- How much is the fare for ...?
- Take me to [...] Street.
- Do you know where the ... is?

Shopping

Asking about Store Hours

- When are you open?
- How late are you open today?
- Are you open on Saturday?

Preliminary Exchanges

- *Hello sir (madam), may I help you?*
- *Can I help you find something?*
- Thank you, I am just looking.
- *I just can't make up my mind.*
- *Can I help you with something?*
- If I can help you, just let me know.
- *Are you looking for something in particular?*
- I am looking for something for my wife.
- I am looking for something for my husband.
- I am looking for something for my children.
- It is a gift.
- Hi, do you sell ...?
- I am looking for a ... Can you help me?
- Would you tell me where the music department is?
- Which floor is the leather goods department on? *On the ground floor (on the mezzanine, on the second floor).*

- Please would you show me ...?
- What kind do you want?
- Where can I find the mirror? There is a mirror over there.
- *The changing rooms are over there.*
- *Only four items are allowed in the dressing room at a time.*
- Is there a public rest room here?
- *Have you decided?*
- *Have you made up your mind?*

Buying Clothes/Shoes

- Please, can you show me some natural silk ties?
- I want to buy a long-sleeved shirt.
- I want the pair of high-heeled shoes I saw in the window.
- Would you please show me the pair in the window?
- What material is it?
- What material is it made of? *Cotton, leather, linen, wool, velvet, silk, nylon, acrylic fiber.*
- What size, please?
- *What size do you need?*
- Is this my size?
- Do you think this is my size?
- Where is the fitting room?
- Does it fit you?
- I think it fits well although the collar is a little tight.
- No, it doesn't fit me.
- May I try a larger size?
- I'll try a smaller size. Would you mind bringing it to me?
- I'll take this one.
- How much is it?
- This is too expensive.
- Oh, this is a bargain!
- I like it.
- May I try this on?
- *In which color?* Navy blue, please.
- Do you have anything to go with this?
- I need a belt/a pair of socks/pair of jeans/pair of gloves. ...
- I need a size 38.
- I don't know my size. Can you measure me?
- Would you measure my waist, please?
- Do you have a shirt to match this?
- Do you have this in blue/in wool/in a larger size/in a smaller size?
- Do you have something a bit less expensive?
- I'd like to try this on. Where is the fitting room?
- How would you like to pay for this? Cash/credit

- *We don't have that in your size/color.*
- *We are out of that item.*
- It's too tight/loose.
- It's too expensive/cheap.
- I don't like the color.
- Is it in the sale?
- Can I have this gift-wrapped?

At the Shoe Store

- A pair of shoes, boots, sandals, slippers, shoelace, sole, heel, leather, suede, rubber, shoehorn.
- *What kind of shoes do you want?*
- I want a pair of rubber-soled shoes/high-heeled shoes/leather shoes/suede slippers/boots.
- I want a pair of lace-up/slip-on shoes good for the rain/for walking.
- *What is your size, please?*
- They are a little tight/too large/too small.
- Would you please show me the pair in the window?
- Can I try a smaller/larger size, please?
- This one fits well.
- I would like some polish cream.
- I need some new laces.
- I need a shoehorn.

At the Post Office

- I need some (first class) stamps, please.
- First class, please.
- Airmail, please.
- I would like this to go express mail.
- I would like this recorded/special delivery.
- I need to send this second-day mail (US).
- Second-class for this, please (UK).
- I need to send this parcel post.
- I need to send this by certified mail.
- I need to send this by registered mail.
- Return receipt requested, please.
- How much postage do I need for this?
- How much postage do I need to send this airmail?
- Do you have any envelopes?
- How long will it take to get there? *It should arrive on Monday.*
- *The forms are over there. Please fill out (UK: fill in) a form and bring it back to me.*

Going to the Theater (UK: Theatre)

- *Sorry, we are sold out tonight.*
- *Sorry, these tickets are non-refundable.*
- *Sorry, there are no tickets available.*
- *Would you like to make a reservation for another night?*
- I would like two seats for tonight's performance, please.
- Where are the best seats you have left?
- Do you have anything in the first four rows?
- Do you have matinees?
- How much are the tickets?
- Is it possible to exchange these for another night?
- Do you take a check/credit cards?
- How long does the show run? *About 2 hours.*
- When does the show close?
- Is there an intermission? *There is an intermission.*
- Where are the rest rooms?
- Where is the cloakroom?
- Is there anywhere we can leave our coats?
- Do you sell concessions?
- How soon does the curtain go up?
- *Did you make a reservation?*
- *What name did you reserve the tickets under?*
- *The usher will give you your program.*

At the Drugstore (UK: Chemist)

- Prescription, tablet, pill, cream, suppository, laxative, sedative, injection, bandage, sticking plasters, cotton wool, gauze, alcohol, thermometer, sanitary towels, napkins, toothpaste, toothbrush, paper tissues, duty chemist.
- Fever, cold, cough, headache, toothache, diarrhea, constipation, sickness, insomnia, sunburn, insect bite.
- I am looking for something for ...
- Could you give me ...?
- Could you give me something for ...?
- I need some aspirin/antiseptic/eye drops/foot powder.
- I need razor blades and shaving foam.
- What are the side effects of this drug?
- Will this make me drowsy?
- Should I take this with meals?

At the Cosmetics Counter

- Soap, shampoo, deodorant, shower gel, hair spray, sun tan cream, comb, hairbrush, toothpaste, toothbrush, make up, cologne water, lipstick, perfume, hair remover, scissors, face lotion, cleansing cream, razor, shaving foam

At the Bookstore/Newsagent's

- I would like to buy a book on the history of the city.
- Has this book been translated into Japanese?
- Do you have Swedish newspapers/magazines/books?
- Where can I buy a road map?

At the Photography Shop

- I want a 36-exposure film for this camera.
- I want new batteries for my camera.
- Could you develop this film?
- Could you develop this film with two prints of each photograph?
- How much does developing cost?
- When will the photographs be ready?
- My camera is not working, would you have a look at it?
- Do you take passport (ID) photographs?
- I want an enlargement of this one and two copies of this other.
- Do you have a 64-megabyte data card to fit this camera?
- How much would a 128-megabyte card be?
- How many megapixels is this one?
- Does it have an optical zoom?
- Can you print the pictures on this CD?

At the Florist

- I would like to order a bouquet of roses.
- *You can choose violets and orchids in several colors.*
- Which flowers are the freshest?
- What are these flowers called?
- Do you deliver?
- Could you please send this bouquet to the NH Abascal Hotel manager at 47 Abascal Street before noon?
- Could you please send this card too?

Paying

- Where is the cash/ATM machine?
- Is there a CashPoint near here?
- How much is that all together?
- *Will you pay cash or by credit card?*
- *Next in line (queue).*
- Could you gift-wrap it for me?
- Can I have a receipt, please?
- Is there a CashPoint near here?
- Can I have a receipt, please?

At the Barber Shop/Salon/Hairdresser

When I was in Boston I went to a salon, and my lack of fluency was responsible for a drastic change in my image for a couple of months so that my wife almost did not recognize me when I picked her up at Logan on one of her multiple visits to New England. I can assure you that I will never forget the word "sideburns"; the stylist, a robust Afro-American lady, drastically cut them before I could recall the name of this insignificant part of my facial hair. To tell you the truth, I did not know how important sideburns were until I did not have them.

If you do not trust an unknown barber/stylist/hairdresser, "just a trim" would be a polite way of avoiding a disaster.

I recommend, before going to have your hair cut, perform a thorough review of your guide so that you get familiar with key words such as: scissors, comb, brush, dryer, shampooing, hair style, hair cut, manicure, dyeing, shave, beard, moustache, sideburns (!) (US), sideboards (UK), fringe, curl, or plait.

Men and Women

- How long will I have to wait?
- *Is the water OK?* It is fine/too hot/too cold.
- My hair is greasy/dry.
- I have dandruff.
- I am losing a lot of hair.
- A shampoo and rinse, please.
- *How would you like it?*
- *Are you going for a particular look?*
- I want a (hair) cut like this.
- Just a trim, please.
- *However you want.*
- *Is it OK?*
- That's fine, thank you.

- How much is it?
- How much do I owe you?
- Do you do highlights?
- I would like a tint, please.

Men
- I want a shave.
- A razor cut, please.
- Just a trim, please.
- Leave the sideburns as they are (!) (UK: sideboards).
- Trim the moustache.
- Trim my beard and moustache, please.
- Toward the back, without any parting.
- I part my hair on the left/in the middle.
- Leave it long.
- Could you take a little more off the top/the back/the sides?
- *How much do you want me to take off?*

Women
- *How do I set your hair?*
- *What hairstyle do you want?*
- I would like my hair dyed/bleached/highlighted.
- *Same color?*
- A little darker/lighter.
- I would like to have a perm (permanent wave).

Cars

As always, begin with key words. Clutch, brake, blinkers (UK: indicators), trunk (UK: boot), tank, gearbox, windshield (UK: windscreen) wipers, (steering) wheel, unleaded gas (UK: petrol), etc., must belong to your fund of knowledge of English, as well as several usual sentences such as:

- How far is the nearest gas (petrol) station? Twenty miles from here.
- In what direction? Northeast/Los Angeles.

At the Gas (UK: Petrol) Station

- Fill it up, please.
- Unleaded, please.
- Could you top up the battery, please?
- Could you check the oil, please?
- Could you check the tire pressures, please?

- *Do you want me to check the spare tire too?* Yes, please.
- Pump number 5, please.
- Can I have a receipt, please?

At the Garage

- My car has broken down.
- What do you think is wrong with it?
- Can you mend a puncture?
- Can you take the car in tow to downtown Boston?
- *I see ..., kill the engine, please.*
- *Start the engine, please.*
- The car goes to the right and overheats.
- *Have you noticed if it loses water/gas/oil?*
- Yes, it's losing oil.
- *Does it lose speed?*
- Yes, and it doesn't start properly.
- I can't get it into reverse.
- The engine makes funny noises.
- Please, repair it as soon as possible.
- I wonder if you can fix it temporarily.
- How long will it take to repair?
- *I am afraid we have to send for spare parts.*
- The car is very heavy on gas.
- I think the right front tire needs changing.
- I guess the valve is broken.
- Is my car ready?
- Have you finished fixing the car?
- Did you fix the car?
- Do you think you can fix it today?
- Could you mend a puncture?
- I think I've got a puncture rear offside.
- The spare's flat as well.
- I've run out of gas.

At the Parking Garage/Structure (UK: Car Park)

- Do you know where the nearest car park is?
- Are there any free spaces?
- How much is it per hour?
- Is the car park supervised?
- How long can I leave the car here?

Renting a Car

- I want to rent a car.
- I want to hire a car.
- *For how many days?*
- *Unlimited mileage?*
- What is the cost per mile?
- Is insurance included?
- *You need to leave a deposit.*

How Can I Get to ...?

- How far is Minneapolis?
- *It is not far. About 12 miles from here.*
- Is the road good?
- *It is not bad, although a bit slow.*
- Is there a toll road between here and Berlin?
- How long does it take to get to Key West?
- I am lost. Could you tell me how I can get back to the turnpike?

Having a Drink (or Two)

Nothing is more desirable than a drink after a hard day of meetings. In such a relaxed situation, embarrassing incidents can happen. Often, there is a difficult counter-question to a simple "Can I have a beer?" such as "would you prefer lager?" or "small, medium or large, sir?" From my own experience, when I was a beginner, I hated counter-questions, and I remember my face flushing when in a pub in London, instead of giving me the beer I asked for, the barman responded with the entire list of beers in the pub. "I have changed my mind; I'll have a Coke instead" was my response to both the "aggression" I suffered from the barman and the embarrassment resulting from my lack of fluency. "We don't serve Coke here, sir." These situations can spoil the most promising evening, So, let us review a some common sentences:

- Two beers please; my friend will pay.
- Two pints of bitter and half a lager, please.
- Where can I find a good place to go for a drink?
- Where can we go for a drink at this time of the evening?
- Do you know any pubs with live music?
- *What can I get you?*
- I'm driving. Just an orange juice, please.
- A glass of wine and two beers, please.

- A gin and tonic.
- A glass of brandy. Would you please warm the glass?
- Scotch, please.
- *Do you want it plain, with water, or on the rocks?*
- Make it a double.
- I'll have the same again, please.
- Two cubes of ice and a teaspoon, please.
- This is on me.
- What those ladies are having is on me.

On the Phone

Many problems start when you lift the receiver. You hear a continuous pur-ring different from the one you are used to in your country or a strange se-quence of rapid pips. Immediately "What the hell am I supposed to do right now?" comes to your mind, and we face one of the most embarras-sing situations for non-fluent speakers. The phone has two added difficul-ties: first, its immediacy and, second, the absence of image ("If I could see this guy I would understand what he was saying"). Do not worry; the pre-liminary exchanges in this conversational scenario are few. Answering ma-chines are another different, and tougher, problem and are out of the scope of this survival guide. Just a tip: Do not hang up. Try to catch what the machine is saying and try it again in case you are not able to follow its instructions. Many doctors, as soon as they hear the unmistakable sound of these devices, terrified, hang up, thinking they are too much for them. Most messages are much easier to understand and less mechanical than those given by "human" (and usually bored) operators.

- Where are the public phones, please?
- Where is the nearest phone booth?
- This telephone is out of order.
- Operator, what do I dial for the USA?
- *Hold on a moment ... the number "1."*
- Would you get me this number please?
- *Dial straight through.*
- What time does the cheap rate begin?
- Do you have any phone cards, please?
- Can I use your cell/mobile phone, please?
- Do you have a phone book (directory)?
- I'd like to make a reverse charge call to Korea.
- I am trying to use my phone card, but I am not getting through.
- Hello, this is Dr. Vida speaking.
- The line is busy.
- There's no answer.
- It's a bad line.

- I've been cut off.
- I would like the number for Dr. Vida on Green Street.
- What is the area code for Los Angeles?
- I can't get through to this number. Would you dial it for me?
- Can you put me through to Spain?

Emergency Situations

- I want to report a fire/a robbery/an accident.
- This is an emergency! We need an ambulance/the police.
- Get me the police, and hurry!

At the Bank

Nowadays, the multitude of credit and debit cards makes this section virtually unnecessary but, in my experience, when things go really wrong, you may need to go to a bank. Fluency disappears in stressful situations so, in case you have to solve a bank problem, review not only this bunch of sentences, but also the entire section in your guide.

- Where can I change money?
- I'd like to change 200 Euros.
- I want to change 1000 Euros into Dollars/Pounds.
- Could I have it in tens, please?
- What's the exchange rate?
- What's the rate of exchange from Euros to Dollars?
- What are the banking hours?
- I want to change this travelers' check.
- Have you received a transfer from Rosario Nadal addressed to Fiona Shaw?
- Can I cash this bearer check?
- I want to cash this check.
- Do I need my ID to cash this bearer check?
- *Go to the cash desk.*
- *Go to counter number 5.*
- May I open a current account?
- Where is the nearest cash machine?
- I am afraid you don't seem to be able to solve my problem. Can I see the manager?
- Who is in charge?
- Could you call my bank in France? There must have been a problem with a transfer addressed to myself.

At the Police Station

- Where is the nearest police station?
- I have come to report a ...
- My wallet has been stolen.
- Can I call my lawyer (UK: solicitor)?
- I have been assaulted.
- My laptop has disappeared from my room.
- I have lost my passport.
- I will not say anything until I have spoken to my lawyer/solicitor.
- I have had a car accident.
- Why have you arrested me? I've done nothing.
- Am I under caution?
- I would like to call my embassy/consulate.

Printing: Krips bv, Meppel, The Netherlands
Binding: Stürtz, Würzburg, Germany